Infectious Diseases of Cattle

Infectious Diseases of Cattle

Authors :

Dr. Rajib Deb
Scientist, Project Directorate on Cattle(ICAR)
Grass Farm Road, Meerut-250 001,UP, India

Dr. Sandip Chakraborty
MVSc (Vet. Microbiology), Veterinary college Bangalore, India

Dr. Umesh Singh
Principle Scientist, Project Directorate on Cattle (ICAR)
Grass Farm Road, Meerut-250 001,UP, India

Dr. Sushil Kumar
Senior Scientist, Project Directorate on Cattle (ICAR)
Grass Farm Road, Meerut-250 001,UP, India

Dr. Arjava Sharma
Director, Project Directorate on Cattle (ICAR)
Grass Farm Road, Meerut-250 001,UP, India

SSPH

SATISH SERIAL PUBLISHING HOUSE
403, Express Tower, Commercial Complex, Azadpur, Delhi-110033 (India)
Phone : 011-27672852, Fax : 91-11-27672046
E-mail :info@satishserial.com, hkjain1975@yahoo.com
Website : www.satishserial.com

Published by :

SATISH SERIAL PUBLISHING HOUSE
403, Express Tower, Commercial Complex, Azadpur, Delhi-110033 (INDIA)
Phone : 011-27672852 Fax : 91-11-27672046
E-mail : info@satishserial.com, hkjain1975@yahoo.com

ISBN 978-93-81226-25-4

Typeset at: Harminder Singh Kharb *for* Laxmi Art Creation
Printed at: Salasar Imaging Systems, Delhi-110035

Dedication

This book is dedicated to the farmers in the Agricultural and Allied Sectors, especially those associated with cattle rearing with a view to uplift their socio-economic condition through transfer of knowledge regarding the management of major infectious diseases of economic importance.

PREFACE

Like human beings, cattle are also affected by a number of diseases or ailments. Every year we lose thousands of healthy animals only because of diseases. This affects our animal productivity very adversely. Since we do not have sufficient facilities to check the spread of these diseases or to carry out proper vaccination programmes, the losses are often very severe. In addition to death, they cause loss of production and frequently a loss of body condition. Unhealthy animals require more food and take longer time for growth than healthy ones, thus causing an indirect economic loss. In general, animals are born free of diseases or parasites. But, they usually acquire these maladies either through contact with diseased animals or due to improper sanitation, feeding, care and management.

The significance of cattle and their contribution to the Indian economy has increased in the present-day context when the impact of rapid industrialisation and mechanisation is taking its toll on the ecological bio-sphere. The contribution of the livestock sector alone is 5.9 % of the total GDP (according to the Government of India's Economic Survey 2001-2002). The major products provided by the livestock sector that aids to the economy of the nation are milk and meat. The figure of milk and meat production in the country provided by cattle and buffalo was 108.5 million tonnes and over 3000 metric tonnes respectively in 2008-2009. So, it is quiet understandable that the occurrence of infectious diseases in cattle hamper the national economy to a greater extent.

Infectious diseases are caused by various bacteria, virus, fungi and parasites. These diseases are spread from animal to animal by contact with diseased animals or their excreta or carcass. Other sources of disease are contaminated feeds, fodder, drinking water and pastures. Many disease causing germs are carried by wind also (as in case of FMD). Further, germs and parasites can be carried by birds, dog, flies, lice, ticks, etc. These disease causing germs or microorganisms enter animal body through various routes like skin, respiratory tract, alimentary canal etc. Once they enter the body, they try to multiply in the body tissues. The body tries to destroy the disease producing agents through the defence system of the body. It consists mainly of the white corpuscles and the disease agents by engulfing them and killing. The antibodies react with the disease causing agents and try to destroy them. This reaction is specific in the sense that the antibody of a particular disease reacts only with the causative agent of that disease. In this process, if the defensive system of the body fails the disease appears.

Strict vigilance against cattle diseases are required as dairy cattle are affected by a variety of diseases. The dairy farmer can prevent disease out-breaks a greater extent by undertaking proper feeding and management programs. Good housing assists in maintaining the health of the herd, whereas judicious feeding not only builds up body resistance to disease but also helps in quick recovery in case of a disease attack.

This book describes the major infectious diseases of cattle along with the diagnostic techniques (conventional to molecular level) and suitable measures undertaken till today to prevent their spread. This book also highlights regarding the major zoonotic diseases transmitted to man from cattle husbandry.

Rajib Deb
Sandip Chakraborty
Umesh Singh
Sushil Kumar
Arjava Sharma

LIST OF FIGURES

1. India ink stained smear revealing the capsule of *B. anthracis*, 5

2. Endospore of *B. anthracis*, 5

3. *B. abortus* revealed by TEM, 11

4. *M. tuberculosis* revealed by ZN staining in tissue section (left) and macrophages (right), 18

5. Haematoxylin and eosin staines smear of IS 900 sequence of *M. paratuberculosis*, 28

6. Non-haemolytic colonies of *P. multocida* on Blood agar, 34

7. Bipolar staining property of *P. multocida*, 34

8. Dark field (a) Shadowed electron and (b) Photomicrographs of *Leptospira* spp., 41

9. *L. monocytogenes* demonstrated by wet mount technique, 44

10. Gangrenous changes in heart muscle affected by *Cl. Chouvei*, 51

11. *Cl. chouvei* in tissue smear stained by gram's staining technique, 51

12. Multiple raised pale tan crusted dermatophyte lesion in bovine skin, 67

13. KOH mounted infected skin showing typical dermatophyte hyphae, 67

14. Immature trophocytes of *R. seeberi* stained by PAS, 69

15. Germ tube formation by *C. albicans* in serum demonstrated by Gram's staining, 70

16. Schematic representation of the pathogenesis of mastitis, 80

17. Structure of foot-and-mouth disease virus, 100

18. Genome map of FMDV, 100

19. Rota virus. A double-capsid particle (left) and a single, inner capsid (right), 120

20. Bullet shaped Rabies virus in its simplest form, 125

21. Leaf like slender form of *T. evansi* with terminal and subterminal kinetoplast, 154

22. Life cycle of *T. annulata*, 161

23. Life cycle of *Babesia* spp., 164

24. Life cycle of *Eimeria* spp., 171

25. Life cycle of *Fasciola* spp., 174

26. Transmission of different species of *Brucella* including *B. abortus* from animals to human, 196

27. Epidemiological cycle of *Leptospira* spp., 201

28. Typical ringworm lesion in human patient, 203

LIST OF TABLES

1. Diseases caused by *Pasteurella* organisms in cattle in India, 32

2. *Leptospira* serovars and their maintenance hosts, 38

3. Diseases caused by different Clostridial spp., 48

4. *Clostridium perfringens* types, major toxins and associated syndromes, 52

5. Changes in milk composition associated with mastitis, 81

6. Relationship between CMT scores and somatic cell count, 83

7. Relationship between SCC linear score (LS) and Somatic cell count (SCC) range, 85

8. Different FMDV serotypes and vaccine strains used for vaccine production, 111

CONTENTS

Dedication .... *v*
Preface .... *vii*
List of Figures .... *ix*
List of Tables .... *xi*

Chapter-1 : Major Bacterial Diseases of Cattle 1
Anthrax 1
Brucellosis 7
Tuberculosis 15
Paratuberculosis (Johne's disease) 24
Pasteurellosis with special reference to Haemorrhagic septicaemia 30
Leptospirosis 37
Listeriosis 42
Clostridial infections 47
References 55

Chapter-2 : Major Fungal Diseases of Cattle 63
Dermatophytoses 64
Rhinosporidiosis 68
Candidiasis 69
References 71

Chapter-3 : Bovine Mastitis 75
Introduction 75
Impact of mastitis in Indian condition 75
Development of the disease 78
Etiological agents 79

Type of mastitis 79
Symptoms 81
Important Diagnostic approaches 81
Prevention and control 87
References 91

Chapter-4 : Major Viral Diseases of Cattle 95
Foot-and-mouth disease (FMD) 96
Infectious bovine rhinotracheitis and infectious pastular vulvovaginitis (IBR-IPV) 112
Rota viral diarrhoea 119
Rabies 124
Blue tongue 132
References 137

Chapter-5 : Major Parasitic Diseases of Cattle 153
Trypanosomiasis/Surra 153
Thileriosis 159
Babesiosis 163
Tick control as a measure for controlling haemoprotozoan diseases like Theileriosis and Babesiosis 169
Coccidiosis in calves 170
Fascioliasis/Liver rot 173
References 177

Chapter-6 : Major Infectious Causes of Abortion in Cattle in India 185
Brucellosis 185
Leptospirosis 186
Listeriosis 187
Campylobacteriosis 187
Salmonellosis 188
Mycoplasmal abortion 188
Mycotic abortion 189
Infectious bovine rhinotracheitis (IBR) 189
Trichomoniasis 190
References 191

Chapter-7 : Major infectious Diseases of Cattle Having Public Health Concern 193
Anthrax 194
Brucellosis 195
Escherichia coli infection 196
Salmonellosis 197
Tuberculosis (T.B) 198
Leptospirosis 199
Listeriosis 202
Ringworm 203
Rabies 204
Fascioliasis 206
References 207

Chapter 1

Major Bacterial Diseases of Cattle

1.1. Anthrax

1.1.1. Introduction

Anthrax, a highly infectious and fatal disease of all warm blooded animals and human, is caused by a relatively large spore-forming rectangular shaped bacterium called *Bacillus anthracis*. The word 'anthrax' arises from the greek word 'coal' due to black coal like cutaneous lesions in human being, especially in people associated with handling animals. Most outbreaks occur in areas where there is previous death of animals due to the disease as the spores are viable for decades. Herbivorous animals are highly susceptible to anthrax, while carnivores, birds and reptiles are resistant.

1.1.2. Etiological agent

The bacterium is a gram positive, non-motile large rod, occurring in short or large chains. The organism is found in two forms *viz.*, the vegetative state and the spore-forming state. The vegetative state, which is the growing, reproducing form found in infected animals, actually causes the disease. If the carcass of an animal died due to anthrax is opened during necropsy, or by scavengers or decay, the vegetative state is exposed to oxygen. This allows the vegetative state to form spores. The spores are highly resistant to disinfectants and the weather and may remain viable in the soil for as many as 50 years. When the spores enter an animal, usually by grazing contaminated vegetation or inhalation, the bacteria revert to the vegetative state. As the organism is aerobic in nature, it consumes 60% of body's oxygen causing sudden death due to acute hypoxia (Parker *et al.*, 2002).

1.1.3. Virulance factors

i) Capsule

ii) Potent exotoxin

The capsule is very unusual in nature as it is polypeptide *i,e.* Poly-D-Glutamate in nature and due to the presence of this capsule the organism can resist phagocytosis. The three important exotoxins are:

i) Protective antigen

ii) Lethal factor

iii) Oedema factor

All these virulence factors are reported in two different plasmids *viz.*, PxO2 that encodes capsule and PxO1 that encodes exotoxins. Normally, non-capsulated strains does not have PxO2 plasmid.

Protective antigen helps in binding of oedema factor and lethal factor. Seven different molecules of protective antigen binds to cell surface in doughnut shaped fashion. Lethal factor is a zinc containing metalloprotease which when released cleaves cellular protein kinase 3, especially in macrophages. It cleaves cellular mitogen activated protein kinase 3 (MAPKK 3) and prevents induction of number of anti-apoptotic genes and thus cause death of macrophages, resulting in loss of capability to phagocytose. Oedema factor is calmodulin dependent adenylate cyclase which increases concentration of cAMP in cell, thus leading to activation of fluid secretion, causing swelling of tissue and ultimately oedema.

1.1.4. Conditions suitable for the occurrence of the disease

Anthrax primarily occurs in alkaline soils with high nitrogen levels caused by decaying vegetation, alternating periods of rain and drought, and temperatures in excess of 60° F. Such areas are referred to as incubator areas where the spores apparently revert to the vegetative form and multiply to infectious levels when optimal environmental conditions occur. Obviously, spores will be found in soils in areas where it has been diagnosed previously. Even in endemic areas, anthrax occurs irregularly, often with many years between outbreaks. It is not well understood why the disease suddenly reappears, but it probably occurs in response to environmental changes. The ideal conditions for reoccurrence of anthrax are increased periods of rainfall and flooding followed by drought. Also, any disturbance of the soil can result in the release of spores.

1.1.5. Clinical signs and post mortem findings

The disease occurs in four different forms *viz.*, peracute, acute, sub acute and chronic forms. Peracute and acute forms are common in cattle. The most common initial sign of anthrax is sudden death. The course of the disease usually is short and varies from one to three days. Animals may exhibit fever, lack of rumination, excitement followed by depression, difficult breathing, uncoordinated movements, convulsions and death during an outbreak. Bloody discharges from the natural body openings and edema in different parts of the body are sometimes observed. Some animals may be saved if antibiotic treatment starts early. In animals that die, bloody discharges from body openings are common. There is rapid decomposition and the carcasses become bloated with gases. Rigor mortis or stiffening is not complete. Haemorrhages in the internal organs and spleenomegaly are common at necropsy.

1.1.6. Human anthrax

Symptoms of the disease vary depending on how the disease was contracted. Usually, there are three forms of anthrax in human. Symptoms usually occur within seven days.

Cutaneous : Most anthrax infections occur when the bacteria enter a cut or abrasion on the skin during handling of contaminated wool, hides, leather or hair products of infected animals. For this reason, the disease is often referred to as "woolsorters disease." Skin infection begins as a raised itchy bump that resembles an insect bite, but within one to two days progresses to a vesicle and then a painless ulcer. Ulcers usually are 1/2 to 1 and1/2 inches in diameter with a characteristic black area in the centre. Other symptoms, such as swollen glands, fever and malaise, often develop after several days, if left untreated. About 20 per cent of untreated cases of cutaneous anthrax results in death, but deaths are rare with appropriate antibiotics.

Inhalation : Initial symptoms may resemble a common cold and include a cough, chills and aches. After several days, however, the symptoms may progress to severe breathing problems and shock. If left untreated, inhalation anthrax usually is fatal.

Intestinal : The intestinal form of anthrax may be contracted following consumption of undercooked, contaminated meat and is characterized by an acute inflammation of the intestinal tract. Initial signs of nausea, loss of appetite, vomiting and fever are followed by abdominal pain, bloody vomition and severe diarrhoea. This form can result in death in 25 to 60 per cent of cases. The relatively short incubation time, coupled with the rapid onset of the disease and quick death, all work to make it unlikely that meat from diseased animals will enter the food chain in any form. Under no circumstances, one should consume meat from infected animals. Spores resist steaming or boiling for five minutes but are killed by autoclaving at 248° F for 20 minutes.

1.1.7. Diagnosis

1.1.7.1. Staining and colony characters

Blood from terminal ear or tail vein are ideal for demonstration of the organisms by polychrome methylene blue staining. The typical 'medusa head' colonies can be demonstrated by isolating the organisms in blood agar. The capsule can be demonstrated by India ink staining.

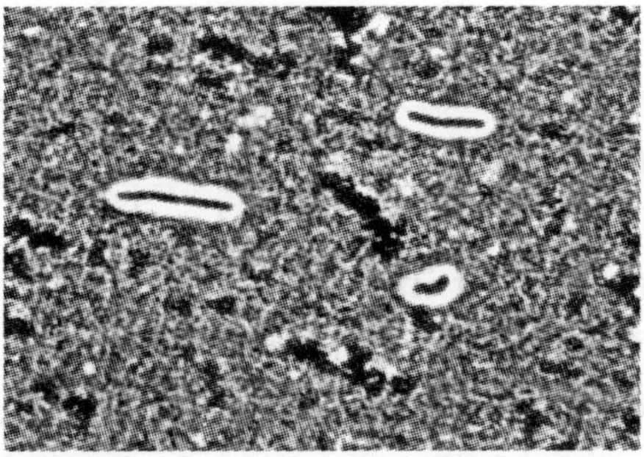

Fig. 1 : India ink stained smear revealing the capsule of *B. anthracis* (http://www.doh.sd.gov)

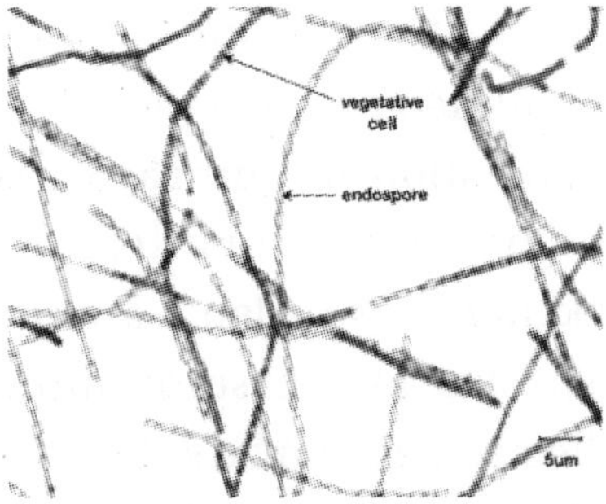

Fig. 2 : Endospore of *B. anthracis* (http://www.faculty.ccbcmd.edu)

1.1.7.2. String of pearl test

This test was first demonstrated by Jansen and Kleymeyer in the year 1953. In this test, tryptose agar (containing 0.5 International Unit of penicillin/ml of medium) is to be inoculated in culture, followed by incubation at 37° C for 3-6 hours. After this, a cover slip is to be placed over the inoculated area and that cover slip is to be examined under microscope wherein organisms are seen as round pearl like instead of normal rod-shaped. On prolonged incubation for 18-24 hours, the organisms may not be seen as they may be killed by penicillin.

1.1.7.3. Ascoli's test

Serological tests like Ascoli's test can be employed for demonstration of the bacterial antigen in decomposed tissue. For this purpose ear or muscle pieces are to be collected in saline, filtered and the filtrate is to be taken in capillary tube. Hyper immune sera is to be added, followed by incubation for 1-2 hours. In positive cases, zone of white precipitate is seen between the filtrate containing the antigen and the hyprimmune sera.

1.1.7.4. Biochemical tests for differentiating *Bacillus anthracis* from anthracoids

Gelatin liquefaction, casein hydrolysis and lecithinase C production are rapid in anthracoids compared to the disease causing organism.

1.1.7.5. Animal innoculation

Guinea pigs are the laboratory animals of choice. Subcutaneous innoculation in guinea pig is done. If animals die within 2-3 days with inflammatory lesion at site of injection and gelatinous subcutaneous oedema appears at the site of innoculation, it may be suspected as a case of anthrax. The spleen or heart blood can be collected and can be subjected to routine staining for anthrax. In mice, pathological material is applied on scarified area at the base of the tail. Positive cases are considered if the animal dies within 2 days.

1.1.7.6. Anthraxin test

For detection of cutaneous anthrax in case of human, anthraxin test can be performed. Surface colonies of *Bacillus anthracis* consists of hair-like curls. These curls are birefringent. The sign of the double refraction is *positive*, with regard to the long axis of these curls, while the sign in cords of colonies of virulent human tubercle bacilli is *negative*. This forms the basis of anthraxin test.

1.1.8. Prevention and control

All the animals in contact with infected animals are to be separated and higher doses of antibiotics like penicillin G is to be given to infected animals. The carcass of an animal suspected of dying from anthrax should never be opened. The discharges and blood are highly infectious to humans and other animals. Opened carcasses will deposit enormous quantities of bacteria on the ground that will sporulate to the long-lasting, protective form. Inhaling bacteria can cause the pulmonary form of the disease in humans. So, great care should be taken to protect anyone who handles carcasses or live animals suspected of having anthrax. All livestock producers should keep a supply of shoulder-length disposable gloves for handling animals that show symptoms of infectious disease. Meat obtained from animals dying of unknown causes or suspected of having anthrax should not be consumed.

Vaccination is another effective means. Institute of Animal Health and Veterinary Biologicals (IAH & VB) produces anthrax spore/Sterne spore vaccine (avirulant live spores are used suspended in 50% glycerol saline). 1 ml of this vaccine should be injected subcutaneously in the caudal skin fold and biurnal vaccination should be followed. All the animals are to be vaccinated one month before the onset of monsoon with Sterne spore vaccine but animals kept for slaughter purpose should not be vaccinated. Precautions should be taken as live spores are used. Needles and syringe should be sterilized and vaccine bottles and vials should be disposed in proper manner. Earlier Pasteur's live vaccine and Carbazoo spore vaccine (spores suspended in 4% saponin) was used. Frequent boosters are required when alum precipitated toxoids are used. At present, recombinant protective antigen based vaccine is in use and confer better immunity.

Disposal of carcass is very important to prevent spreading of disease. Dragging of carcass is prohibited. Deep burial or incineration after applying quick lime is suggested. 5% quick lime, 0.5% sodium hypochlorite, 3% hydrogen per oxide, 10% formalin, peracetic acid and glutaraldehyde are sporicidal in nature and can be used for decontamination of equipments.

1.2. Brucellosis

1.2.1. Introduction

Brucellosis is an important re-emerging zoonosis with a worldwide distribution. Brucellosis is an important re-emerging infectious disease and has undoubtedly evolved as a disease since man first domesticated animals. Brucellosis was recognized as a clinical entity from the times of Crimean war. This disease was fully elucidated by Sir David Bruce, Hughes, and Zammit working in Malta. Bang discovered *Brucella abortus*, the cause of abortion in cattle and undulant fever in human beings. Bovine brucellosis, caused by the bacterium *Brucella abortus*, is an economically important cause of abortions in cattle. The disease is still an uncontrolled serious public health problem in many developing countries including India. Brucellosis in India is yet a very common but often neglected disease. Isolated cases of non-terrestrial brucellosis and continuing transmission from wild animals have raised important epidemiological issues. Laboratory testing is indispensable for diagnosis. Advances in newer rapid, sensitive, and specific testing methodologies and alternate treatment strategies are urgently needed. Safe and effective vaccine in human is not yet available. Increased public awareness through health education programmes and safe livestock practices forms the basis of prevention (Mantur and Amarnath 2008).

1.2.2. Etiological agent

Brucellae belong to á–2 subdivision of *proteobacteria*. They are Gram-negative, partially acid fast, aerobic, facultative intracellular coccobacilli or short rods. They are oxidase, catalase, nitrate reductase and urease positive. The genome contains two circular chromosomes of 2.1 Mb and 1.5 Mb except *B.suis* biovar 3 which has a single chromosome of 3.1 Mb. There are two types of smooth lipopolysaccharide (SLPS) surface antigens, designated A and M. A antigen predominates in *B. abortus* and *B. suis*, while M is the major antigen in *B. melitensis*. Numerous outer and inner membrane, cytoplasmic, and periplasmic proteins have also been characterized.

1.2.3. Pathogenesis

Brucellae can enter mammalian hosts through skin abrasions or cuts, the conjunctiva, the respiratory tract, and the gastrointestinal tract. In the gastrointestinal tract, the organisms are phagocytosed by lymphoepithelial cells of gut-associated lymphoid tissue, from which they gain access to the submucosa. Organisms are rapidly ingested by polymorphonuclear leukocytes, which generally fail to kill them and are also phagocytosed by macrophages. The organism ultimately localize in lymph nodes, spleen, mammary glands, joints, kidneys and bone marrow, being carried by the macrophages (Elsbach 1980).

In macrophages, brucellae inhibit fusion of phagosomes and lysosomes and replicate within compartments that contain components of endoplasmic reticulum via a process facilitated by the type IV secretion system. If unchecked by macrophage microbicidal mechanisms, the bacteria destroy their host cells and infect additional cells. Brucellae can also replicate extracellularly in host tissues (Pizarro-Cerda *et al.,* 1998). In cattle, *Brucella* organisms bypass the most effective host defenses by targeting embryonic and trophoblastic tissue. In cells of these tissues, the bacteria grow not only in the phagosome but also in the cytoplasm and the rough endoplasmic reticulum. In the absence of effective intracellular microbicidal mechanisms, these tissues permit exuberant bacterial growth, which leads to fetal death and abortion. The presence of erythritiol in the placenta may further enhance growth of brucellae (Anderson *et al.,* 1986).

1.2.4. Epidemiology

In animals, infection usually occurs by ingestion and through mucous membranes, but *B. abortus* can be transmitted through broken skin. Although the mammary gland is usually colonized during the course of an infection, it can also be infected by direct contact, with subsequent shedding of the organisms in the milk. *In utero* infections also occur. Venereal transmission seems to be uncommon. Transmission by artificial insemination is reported to occur when contaminated semen is deposited in the uterus but not in the midcervix. *B. abortus* can spread through fomites including feed and water. In conditions of high humidity, low temperatures, and no sunlight, these organisms can remain viable for several months in water, aborted fetuses, manure, wool, hay, equipment and clothes. *Brucella* species can withstand drying, particularly when organic material is present and can survive in dust and soil. Survival is longer when the temperature is low, particularly when it is below freezing. Animals may transmit *Brucella* organisms to human during septic abortion, during slaughter, and through their milk. Brucellosis is rarely, if ever, transmitted from person to person. The incidence of human disease is thus closely related to the prevalence of infection in ruminants like cattle, and to practices that allow exposure of humans to potentially infected animals or their products. The organism is highly infectious in laboratory settings as well.

1.2.5. Clinical signs and post-mortem findings

In previously unexposed and unvaccinated cattle, *B. abortus* spreads rapidly and abortion storms are common. The abortion rate varies from 30% to 80%. In herds where this organism has become endemic, only sporadic symptoms occur and cows may abort their first pregnancies. The abortion usually occurs during the second half of gestation. Some calves are born alive but weak, and may die soon after birth. There may be retention of placenta and secondary metritis. Lactation may be decreased. After the first abortion, subsequent pregnancies are generally normal. However, cows may shed the organism in milk and uterine discharges. Epididymitis, seminal vesiculitis, orchitis or testicular abscesses are sometimes seen in bulls. Infertility occurs occasionally in both sexes, due to metritis or orchitis/ epididymitis. Hygromas, particularly on the leg joints, are a common symptom in some tropical countries. Arthritis can develop in some long-term infections. Systemic signs do not usually occur in uncomplicated infections, and deaths are rare except in the fetus or newborn. Infections in nonpregnant females are usually asymptomatic.

At necropsy, granulomatous inflammatory lesions may be present in the reproductive tract, udder, supramammary lymph nodes, other lymphoid tissues, and sometimes in the joints and synovial membranes. Mild to severe endometritis may be seen after an abortion. The placenta is usually thickened and edematous, and may have exudate on its surface. The intercotyledonary region is typically leathery, with a wet appearance and focal thickening. The regional lymph nodes can be enlarged, and the mammary gland may contain lesions. Some aborted fetuses appear normal; others are autolyzed or have variable amounts of subcutaneous edema and bloodstained fluid in the body cavities. The liver may be enlarged and discolored, and the lungs may exhibit fibrous pleuritis and pneumonia. In bulls, one or both sacs of the scrotum may be swollen due to orchitis, epididymitis or abscesses. The tunica vaginalis may be thickened and fibrous, and adhesions may be present. Hygromas may be found at slaughter in both sexes on the knees, stifles, hock, angle of the haunch, and between the nuchal ligament and the primary thoracic spines.

1.2.6. Diagnosis

Brucellosis should be considered in all abortions, particularly when there are multiple late-term abortions in the herd. The disease in cattle should be differentiated from trichomoniasis, vibriosis, leptospirosis, listeriosis, infectious bovine rhinotracheitis and various mycoses.

1.2.6.1. Detection of organism in smears

Microscopic examination of smears stained with the Stamp's modification of the Ziehl-Neelsen method can be useful for a presumptive diagnosis, particularly if the direct examination is supported by serology. *Brucell*a species are not truly acid-fast, but they are resistant to decolorization by weak acids, and stain red against a blue background. Brucellae are coccobacilli or short rods, usually arranged singly but sometimes in pairs or small groups. This test is not definitive. Other organisms such as *Chlamydophila abortus* and *Coxiella burnetii* can resemble *Brucella*. For this reason, immunostaining is sometimes used to identify *Brucella* in smears. Even transmission electron microscopy (TEM) is conducted to demonstrate the organism.

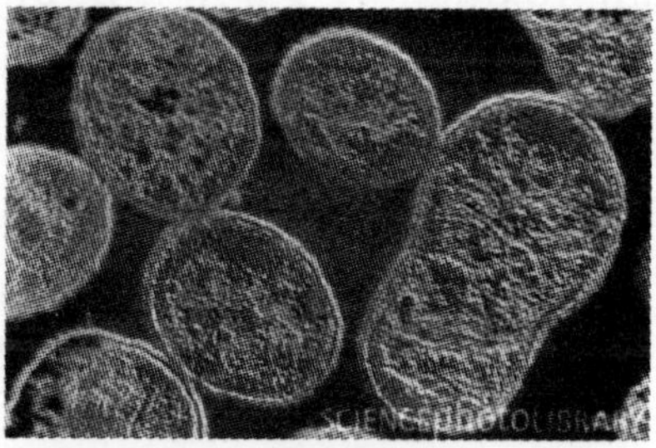

Fig. 3 : *B. abortus* revealed by TEM (http://www. sciencephoto.com)

1.2.6.2. Cultural examination

Bacteriological examination is the absolute proof of *Brucella* infection and its epidemiological studies to determine the species and biotype of the isolated strain. Therefore, bacteriologic examination on aborted fetuses or placentas should be undertaken whenever possible. Vaginal discharges, if taken shortly after parturition and milk samples are suitable for cultures. Selective media like serum dextrose agar or tryptose agar make it possible to isolate the organisms from contaminated specimens. Bacteriological examination of aborted material is time consuming, laborious, costly and cannot routinely be used as a diagnostic procedure in developing countries like India (Chakraborty 2012). A definitive diagnosis can be made if *B. abortus* is cultured from an animal. *Brucella* spp. can be isolated on a variety of plain media, or selective media such as Farrell's medium or Thayer-Martin's modified medium. Enrichment techniques can also be used. *Brucella* colonies usually become visible after two days growth and after four days of incubation, the colonies appear to be round and approximately 1-2 mm in diameter with smooth margins. When the plates are viewed in daylight through a transparent medium, the colonies are transluscent and a pale honey colour. From above, they are convex and pearly white. Smooth (S) *Brucella* cultures can dissociate to rough (R) forms. These colonies are much less transparent and become more granular and dull. In crystal violet staining, rough colonies stain red and smooth colonies stain pale yellow.

1.2.6.3. Serological tests

Serology can be used for a presumptive diagnosis of brucellosis, or to screen herds. Serological tests used to test individual cattle and herds include the buffered *Brucella* antigen tests (rose bengal test and buffered plate agglutination test), complement fixation, indirect or competitive enzyme-linked immunosorbent assays (ELISAs) or the fluorescence polarization assay. Other serological tests include rivanol precipitation, acidified antigen procedures and the serum agglutination test (tube or microtiter test). Supplemental tests such as complement fixation or rivanol precipitation are often used to clarify the results from plate or card agglutination tests. Buffered Plate Anigen Test (BPAT) is having the highest sensitivity for screening cattle. Sensitivity and specificity of more than 2 screening tests can be estimated simultaneously without a gold standard by use of Bayesian techniques (Fosgate *et al.*, 2002). ELISAs or the *Brucella* milk ring test (BRT) can be used to screen herds by detecting antibodies in milk. In vaccinated cattle, the native hapten -based gel precipitation tests (gel diffusion or radial immunodiffusion tests) are sometimes used to distinguish vaccinated animals from infected animals. Standard Tube Aggluitination Test (SAT) remains the most popular and yet used worldwide diagnostic tool. SAT measures the total quantity of agglutinating antibodies (IgM and IgG), and the quantity of specific IgG is determined by 2-mercaptoethanol (2ME). SAT titres above 1:160 are considered diagnostic in conjunction with a compatible clinical presentation. In endemic areas, a titre of 1:320 as cut-off may make the test more specific. The of type of antibody is important, as IgG antibodies are considered a better indicator of active infection and the rapid fall in the level of IgG antibodies is said to be prognostic of successful therapy. The studies by Mantur *et al.* (2006) have shown persistence of various levels of SAT antibodies in many clinically cured patients. This emphasizes the over diagnosis and diagnostic challenges faced in an area where typhoid, malaria, tuberculosis and rheumatoid arthritis clinically mimic human brucellosis, thereby denying patients having access to specific therapy. Coombs test that detects incomplete antibodies and immunocapture-agglutination tests have shown similar performances with higher sensitivity and specificity in the diagnosis. *Brucella* IgM and IgG lateral flow and latex agglutination assays have been found to be rapid and simple along with high sensitivity and specificity in culture confirmed cases. These tests are ideal for use as field tests. Animal inoculation is rarely used to isolate *B. abortus*, but may be necessary if other techniques fail. Guinea pigs or mice are the animals of choice in such instances.

1.2.6.4. Molecular tools

Polymerase chain reaction (PCR) techniques and other genetic techniques likerestriction fragment length polymorphism or Southern blotting are available in some laboratories. Similar tests are also used to diagnose *B. abortus* infections in species other than cattle, but each test must be validated in that species. The detection of polymorphism of natural resistance associated macrophage protein1 (NRAMP1/SLC11A1) gene that has potential role in conferring innate resistance against *B. abortus* infection by PCR-RFLP studies have also been carried out in recent past (Kumar *et al.*, 2011).

1.2.6.5. Brucellin test

Brucellin allergic skin test can be used to test unvaccinated cattle for *B. abortus*. This test is performed by injecting the allergen intradermally into the caudal fold, the skin of the flank, or the side of the neck.

1.2.7. Prevention and control

Bovine brucellosis is usually introduced into a herd in an infected animal, but it can also enter in semen from infected bulls and on fomites. In endemic areas, vaccinated calves or non-pregnant heifers are the best herd additions in uninfected herds. Any pregnant or fresh cows should come from brucellosis-free areas or herds, and should be seronegative. Herd additions should be isolated for approximately a month and re-tested for *B. abortus* before they are added to the herd. Eradication can be accomplished by quarantine of infected herds, vaccination, test-and-slaughter techniques, various forms of surveillance and tracebacks. Any area exposed to infected animals and their discharges should be thoroughly cleaned and disinfected. Infections in other species are generally prevented by controlling *B. abortus* in its maintenance hosts.

Two *B. abortus* vaccines, Strain 19 and RB51, can be used to control this disease in endemic areas, or used as part of an eradication program. Routine vaccination is often done in calves to minimize the production of persistent antibodies that can interfere with serological tests. In the U.S., RB51 has largely replaced Strain 19. RB51 is less likely to induce persistent antibodies, and it is safer for humans. However, since both the vaccines are live, they can cause abortions in pregnant cattle and adverse effects in humans. These two vaccine strains (*B. abortus* strains S19 and RB51) can be distinguished from field strains by their growth characteristics and sensitivity to antibiotics which can aid to diagnosis.

1.3. Tuberculosis

1.3.1. Introduction

Bovine tuberculosis is a chronic bacterial disease of cattle that occasionally affects other species of mammals. This disease is a significant zoonosis that can spread to humans, typically by the inhalation of aerosols or the ingestion of unpasteurized milk. In developed countries, eradication programs have reduced or eliminated tuberculosis in cattle, and human disease is now rare but the disease is still prevalent in developing country like India, both in cattle as well as human population. Reservoirs in wildlife can make complete eradication difficult. Bovine tuberculosis is still common in less developed countries, and severe economic losses can occur from livestock deaths, chronic disease and trade restrictions. In some situations, this disease may also be a serious threat to endangered species.

1.3.2. Etiological agent

Bovine tuberculosis results from infection by *Mycobacterium bovis*, a Gram positive, acid-fast bacterium in the *Mycobacterium tuberculosis* complex of the family Mycobacteriaceae. Other members of the *M. tuberculosis* complex, previously considered to be *M. bovis,* have been accepted as new species despite identical 16s RNA sequences and over 99.9% identity of their genome sequences. These include *M. caprae*, a primary pathogen of goats and *M. pinnipedii*, a pathogen of fur seals and sea lions. These two new species are known to be zoonotic. In central Europe, *M. caprae* has been identified as a common cause of bovine tuberculosis (Prodinger *et al.*, 2005). Disease caused by *M. caprae* is not considered to be substantially different from that caused by *M. bovis*.

1.3.3. Epidemiology

M. bovis can be transmitted by the inhalation of aerosols, by ingestion, or through breaks in the skin. The importance of these routes varies between species. Bovine tuberculosis is usually maintained in cattle populations, but a few other species can become reservoir hosts. Most species are considered to be spillover hosts. Populations of spillover hosts do not maintain *M. bovis* indefinitely in the absence of maintenance hosts, but may transmit the infection between their members or to other species for a certain period of time. Some spillover hosts can become maintenance hosts if their population density is high. Cattle shed *M. bovis* in respiratory secretions, faeces and milk, and sometimes in the urine, vaginal secretions or semen. Large numbers of organisms may be shed in the terminal stages of infection. Asymptomatic and anergic carriers occur. In most cases, *M. bovis* is transmitted between cattle in aerosols during close contact. Infection through ingestion is particularly important in calves that nurse from infected cows. Cutaneous, genital, and congenital infections have been seen but are rare. All infected cattle may not transmit the disease.

1.3.4. Clinical signs and post mortem lesions

Early infections are often asymptomatic. In the late stages, common symptoms include progressive emaciation, a low-grade fluctuating fever, weakness and inappetence. Animals with pulmonary involvement usually have a moist cough that is worse in the morning, during cold weather or exercise, and may have dyspnoea or tachypnea. In the terminal stages, animals may become extremely emaciated and develop acute respiratory distress. In some animals, the retropharyngeal or other lymph nodes enlarge and may rupture and drain. Greatly enlarged lymph nodes can also obstruct blood vessels, airways, or the digestive tract. If the digestive tract is involved, intermittent diarrhoea and constipation may be seen. In maintenance hosts other than cattle, the prevalence of infection and the severity of the disease vary with the species.

At post-mortem, tubercles are found in the lymph nodes, particularly those of the head and thorax. They are also common in the lung, spleen, liver and the surfaces of body cavities. In disseminated cases, multiple small granulomas may be found in numerous organs. Lesions are sometimes found on the female genitalia, but are rare on the male genitalia. In countries with good control programs, infected cattle typically have few lesions at necropsy. Most of these lesions are found in the lymph nodes associated with the respiratory system. However, small lesions can often be discovered in the lungs of these animals if the tissues are sectioned. When calves are exposed to the tuberculosis bacteria in the milk, the most common lesions are noted in the lymph nodes at the junction of the neck and head around the throat. The main sign may be swelling of these nodes. The primary lesions in calves, however, are most frequently located in the lymph nodes along the intestinal tract (Kirk 2002).

1.3.5. Diagnosis

Tuberculosis can be difficult to diagnose based only on the clinical signs. The disease should be differentiated from contagious bovine pleuropneumonia, *Pasteurella* or *Corynebacterium pyogenes* pneumonia, aspiration pneumonia (which is often secondary to chronic wasting disease, traumatic pericarditis, caseous lymphadenitis or melioidosis in small ruminants and chronic aberrant liver fluke infestation.

1.3.5.1. Presumptive diagnosis and staining

A presumptive diagnosis can be made by histopathology and/or the microscopic demonstration of acid-fast bacilli. Direct smears from clinical samples or tissues may be stained with the Ziehl-Neelsen

(ZN) stain, a fluorescent acid-fast stain or immunoperoxidase techniques.

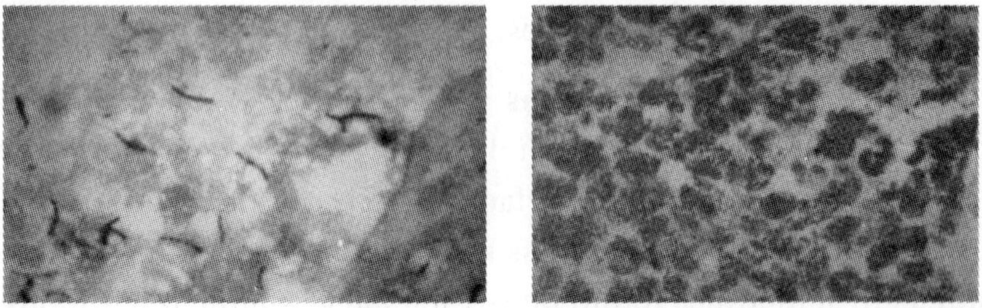

Fig. 4 : *M. tuberculosis* revealed by ZN staining in tissue section (left) and macrophages (right)
(http://www.scientissolutions.com, http://www.pathologyoutlines.com).

1.3.5.2. Cultural examination

Culture is still recognised as the gold standard for diagnosis of infection with *M. bovis* (Cousins and Florisson 2005). Prescapular lymph gland is the most appropriate specimens for isolation of *M. bovis* from infected cattle. Swollen lymph node especially of the head, and discharging lymph node abscesses are important clinical signs of tuberculosis infection in animals. Thus lymph glands can be recommended as a preferred specimen for confirmation of diagnosis of bovine tuberculosis. Faeces and milk are considered as important media for transmission of bovine tuberculosis. Even blood can be used as specimen for detection of tuberculosis in cattle (Srivastava *et al.,* 2008). For primary isolation, the sediment derived by centrifugation of the processed clinical specimen is usually inoculated on to a set of solid egg-based media, such as Lowenstein–Jensen, Coletsos base or Stonebrinks. These media should contain either pyruvate or pyruvate and glycerol. An agar-based medium such as Middlebrook 7H10 or 7H11 or blood based agar medium may also be used (Cousins *et al.,* 1989). Cultures are incubated for a minimum of 8 weeks and maximum upto 10–12 weeks at 37°C with or without CO2. The media should be in tightly closed tubes to avoid desiccation. Slopes are examined for macroscopic growth at intervals during the incubation period. When growth is visible, smears are prepared and stained by the Ziehl–Neelsen technique. Growth of *M. bovis* generally occurs within 3–6 weeks of incubation depending on the media used. Liquid culture systems are used routinely in some hospital and veterinary laboratories; in these systems growth is measured by radiometric or fluorometric methods.

1.3.5.3. Tests for detecting cell mediated immunity

1.3.5.3.1. Tuberculin test

It is a prescribed test for international trade. It involves intradermal injection of *M. bovis* purified protein derivative (PPD) tuberculin and the subsequent detection of a swelling (delayed hypersensitivity) at the site of injection three days later. It has been in use since the early 1900s and is still the tool of choice for most bovine tuberculosis eradication and control programmes. The tuberculin test is the only test for tuberculosis in cattle prescribed by the World Organisation for Animal Health (OIE).

1.3.5.3.2. Gamma interferon assay

This is an alternative test for international trade. In this test, the release of a lymphokine gamma interferon (IFN-ã) is measured in a whole-blood culture system. The assay is based on the release of IFN-ã from sensitised lymphocytes during an incubation period of 16-24 hours with specific antigen *viz.*, tuberculin. The test makes use of the comparison of IFN-g production following stimulation with avian and bovine PPD. The detection of bovine IFN-ã is carried out with a sandwich ELISA that uses two monoclonal antibodies to bovine gamma-interferon. It is however recommended that the blood samples must be transported to the laboratory and the assay set up as soon as possible, but not later than the day after blood collection. In some areas, especially where 'non specificity' is prevalent, some concerns about the accuracy have been expressed. However, because of the IFN-ã test capability of detecting early infections, the use of both tests in parallel allows detection of a greater number of infected animals before they become a source of infection for other animals as well as a source of contamination of the environment (Gormley *et al.*, 2006).

1.3.5.3.3. Lymphocyte proliferation assay

This type of *in-vitro* assay compares the reactivity of peripheral blood lymphocytes to tuberculin PPD (PPDB) and a PPD from *Mycobacterium avium* (PPD-A). The assay can be performed on whole blood or on purified lymphocytes from peripheral blood samples. These tests endeavour to increase the specificity of the assay by removing the response of lymphocytes to cross-reactive antigens associated with non-pathogenic species of mycobacteria to which the animal may have been exposed. Results are usually analysed as the value obtained in response to PPD-B minus the value obtained in response to PPDA. The B–A value must then be above a cut-off point that can be altered in order to maximise either specificity or sensitivity of the diagnosis. The assay has scientific value, but is not used for routine diagnosis because the test is time-consuming and the logistics and laboratory execution are complicated as it requires long incubation times and the use of radio-active nucleotides.

1.3.5.4. Tests for humoral response

1.3.5.4.1. Enzyme-linked Immuno Sorbent Assay (ELISA)

The ELISA appears to be the most suitable of the antibody-detection tests and can be a complement, rather than an alternative, to tests based on cellular immunity. It may be helpful in anergic cattle and deer. An advantage of the ELISA is its simplicity, but sensitivity is limited mostly because of the late and irregular development of the humoral immune response in cattle during the course of the disease. Specificity is also poor in cattle when complex antigens such as tuberculin or *M. bovis* culture filtrates are used. However, a comparison of antibody levels to PPD-B and PPD-A has been shown to be useful in increasing specificity in the ELISA (Griffin *et al.*, 1993).

1.3.5.4.2. Florescent Polarization Assay (FPA)

The FPA is based on the principle that an antigen bound in an immunocomplex will have a higher polarisation value than free antigen. The principal advantage of FPA is that no separation of bound from free antigen is required. The entire assay is performed in solution in a single tube, with no precipitation or washing steps (Dandliker *et al.*, 1973).

1.3.5.4.3. Multi-antigen Print Immunoassay (MAPIA)

The MAPIA consists of a cocktail of antigens applied by micro-aerosolisation to nitrocellulose membranes in narrow bands. Strips cut perpendicular to the antigen bands are subject to a blocking step and incubated with serum samples, and this is followed by immunodetection using standard chromogenic methods (Lyashchenko *et al.*, 2000).

1.3.5.4.4. Chembio rapid test

This test is based upon the detection, in infected animals, of antibodies to a set of recombinant tuberculosis (TB) antigens. The format is a proprietary lateral flow test that uses a drop of blood and gives a visual result within 15 minutes (Greenwald *et al.*, 2003).

1.3.5.5. Nucleic acid recognition methods

Rapid identification of isolates to the level of *M. tuberculosis* complex can be made by Gen Probe TB complex DNA probe or polymerase chain reaction (PCR) targeting 16S and 23S rRNA, the insertion sequences IS*6110* and IS*1081*, and genes coding for *M.-tuberculosis*-complex-specific proteins, such as MPB70 and the 38 kDa antigen b have been used. Specific identification of an isolate as *M. bovis* can be made using PCR targeting a mutation at nucleotide positions 285 in the *oxy*R gene, 169 in the *pncA* gene, 675/756/1311/1410 and 1450 of the *gyr*B gene and presence or absence of regions of difference (Parsons *et al.*, 2002). Alternatively molecular typing techniques, such as spoligotyping will identify *M. bovis* isolates and provide some molecular-typing information on the isolate that is of epidemiological value.

PCR has recently been used for the diagnosis of tuberculosis in animals. A number of commercially available kits and various in-house methods have been evaluated for the detection of the *M. tuberculosis* complex in fresh and fixed tissues. Amplified products can be analysed by hybridisation with probes or by gel electrophoresis. Commercial kits and the in-house methods, in fresh, frozen or boric acid-preserved tissues, have shown variable and less than satisfactory results in interlaboratory comparisons (Noredhoek *et al.*, 1996). False-positive and falsenegative results, particularly in specimens containing low numbers of bacilli, have reduced the reliability of this test. Although direct PCR can produce a rapid result, it is recommended that culture be used in parallel to confirm a viable *M. bovis* infection.

A variety of DNA-fingerprinting techniques has been developed that can distinguish between different strains of *M. bovis* and helps in recognizing patterns of origin, transmission and spread of *M. bovis* (Durr *et al.*, 2000). The most widely used method is spoligotyping which allows the differentiation of strains inside each species belonging to the *M. tuberculosis* complex, including *M. bovis*, and can also distinguish *M. bovis* from *M. tuberculosis* (Kamerbeek *et al.*, 1997). The genome of *M. bovis* has been sequenced which has contributed to improved methods of genetic fingerprinting and to the development of PCR assays that define the subspecies of the *M. tuberculosis* complex.

1.3.6. Prevention and control

Bovine tuberculosis can be controlled by either test-and-slaughter or test-and-segregation methods. Affected herds are re-tested periodically to eliminate cattle that may shed the organism. For this purpose, the tuberculin test is generally used. Infected herds are usually quarantined, and animals that have been in contact with reactors are traced. Only test-and-slaughter techniques are guaranteed to eradicate tuberculosis from domesticated animals. Once eradication is nearly complete, slaughter surveillance, with tracing of infected animals, may be a more efficient use of resources. Sanitation and disinfection may reduce the spread of the agent within the herd. *M. bovis* is relatively resistant to disinfectants and requires long contact times for inactivation. Effective disinfectants include 5% phenol, iodine solutions with a high concentration of available iodine, glutaraldehyde and formaldehyde. In environments with low concentrations of organic material, 1% sodium hypochlorite with a long contact time is also effective. *M. bovis* is also susceptible to moist heat of 121°C (250°F) for a minimum of 15 minutes. Rodent control is also be advisable on affected farms. The occurrence of *M. bovis* in wildlife reservoir hosts complicates eradication efforts. Transmission from wild life reservoirs can be decreased by culling programme. However, each situation must be assessed individually as culling may have unanticipated effects such as increasing the dispersal of the remaining members of a species. Prohibition of supplemental feeding and baiting can decrease transmission at feeding areas. Barriers can be used around hay storage areas to prevent wildlife access. In addition, biosecurity measures on farms decrease interactions between wildlife and domesticated animals.

At present the only available vaccine against *M. bovis* infections is bacille-Calmette-Guerin (BCG), which is a live attenuated strain of *M. bovis*. This has shown variable efficacy in cattle trials. Trials have been conducted on a number of other vaccines, but none has been shown to induce a superior protection to BCG. The efficacy of BCG has been shown to vary in a similar manner to that reported for humans. Before taking up a vaccination programme, the vaccination schedule must be optimised for local conditions. Typical dosage should be from 10^4 to 10^6 colony-forming units that has to be given subcutaneously. Vaccine should be based on the standard reference strain, BCG Pasteur or Danish (World Health Organization 1994). It is important to recognise that use of vaccine will compromise tuberculin skin tests or other immunological tests relying on the use of tuberculin as diagnostic antigen. Thus, vaccination in cattle should not be used in areas where control or trade measures based on such testing are in operation. However, significant progress has been made in the development of so-called DIVA antigens that allow the differentiation of BCG vaccinated from *M. bovis* infected animals, particularly when used in the gamma-interferon test. Such antigens are based on the use of antigens that are encoded on *M. bovis* gene regions that are deleted in BCG (such as ESAT-6 and CFP-10), that are under-expressed in some BCG strains (such as MPB83), or are not secreted by BCG (such as Rv3615c) (Vordermeier *et al.*, 2001; Sidders *et al.*, 2008).

1.4. Paratuberculosis (Johne's disease)

1.4.1. Introduction

Paratuberculosis (Johne's disease) is a chronic infectious dreaded disease of domestic animals though some wild ruminants and laboratory animals are also susceptible to the same. Johne's disease causes huge production losses and has high impact on animal industry (Deb *et al.*, 2011). It is an enzootic disease on the B list of the Office des International Epizootes ('OIE'). The disease is prevalent in both domestic and exotic cattle and is caused by *Mycobacterium avium sub species paratuberculosis* (Map), is ubiquitous and distributed throughout the world including India. No effective therapeutics or vaccines are available ill date and early detection along with good management practices is the only way to control paratuberculosis.

1.4.2. Etiological agent

The identification of Map is attributed to F.W. Twort, who in 1912 showed that the causative agent of the disease could be cultivated in vitro. The organism is acid as well as alcohol fast, slow growing fastidious bacterium and requires exogenous mycobactin J when grown in vitro. This organism has also been reported to be associated with cases of Crohn's disease, a chronic fatal multifactorial inflammatory bowel disease in humans.

1.4.3. Epidemiology

Bacteria can be passed to a cow's unborn foetus and is excreted in the faeces and milk of infected adult cattle. Transmission to calf can occur before birth, or as a result of nursing infected dam, or as a result of ingesting contaminated faecal material on teats and hair as well as feed and water. New born calves below the age of one month are most susceptible to infection. As the calves grow older, they become more resistant to infection. In an infected newborn, the bacteria invade the lining of the intestinal epithelium where they multiply slowly for 2 or more years and as a result sub clinical infection develops. The organism can be shed in the faeces and milk of the infected animal before they develop clinical signs which makes sub clinically infected animal an important source of infection. Clinical signs of the disease appear only in the adult cattle and is often associated with some forms of stress, such as calving or crowding. Clinically infected cattle spread the disease through faeces which is considered to be a threat to the herd. Cattle can shed organisms as long as 18 months after developing clinical signs. The bacteria don't multiply in the environment, but can survive in the soil and water for more than a year because of resistance to heat, cold and drying.

1.4.4. Clinical signs and affect of the disease

Clinical signs in an infected cow commonly appear within a few weeks after calving. Diseased cattle continue to eat, but have constant or recurring bouts of diarrhoea. Some cattle may appear to recover temporarily, but will relapse. Typically, less than 1 percent of an infected herd may show clinical signs of the disease in a given year. The common history in an infected dairy herd is a 5 to 20 percent reduction in milk production and an occasional cow with diarrhoea and weight loss. For every clinical animal, there are likely to be 15 to 25 sub clinical animals in the herd. Production losses in affected herds result from premature culling and reduced milk production. In addition, the poor body condition in culled open cows further widens the economic spread between prices of culled cows and costs of heifer replacement.

In adult cattle, the bacteria cause enteritis, an inflammation of the small intestine that becomes thickened and corrugated. Poor absorption of nutrients occurs and watery diarrhoea develops. Even though the animal has a good appetite, the animal rapidly loses weight, becomes weak and emaciated with a bottle jaw, and either dies or is culled. Cattle rapidly become emaciated. However, the wasting often progresses over a few months.

1.4.5. Diagnosis

The past decade has witnessed the development and commercialization of multiple accurate and cost-effective diagnostic tests for paratuberculosis that are based on detection of antibodies to *M paratuberculosis* in serum or milk or detection of the etiologic agent in faeces from specific cattle or the farm environment by conventional bacterial culture, bacterial culture by use of an automated liquid culture system, or genetic detection systems *viz.*, PCR assays. Although the availability of several tests for paratuberculosis provides options for detection and control of the disease, it also causes confusion for practitioners and producers with regard to the test that should be used for a specific purpose.

1.4.5.1. Bacterial culture of faecal sample

Faecal samples can be collected from areas in which cattle from a herd commingle. Such samples should be collected in accordance with Uniform Program Standards and are cultured on solid HEY agar medium, and appropriate testing is conducted to confirm the Map isolates (USDA-APHIS 2006). Testing of faecal samples obtained from individual cattle can also include bacterial culture by use of any commercial liquid culture system. Similar to isolates cultured by use of solid HEY agar, isolates cultured by use of liquid culture systems should be subjected to appropriate testing for confirmation. Bacterial culture can also be performed on pooled faecal samples obtained from several cattle in a herd. It is recommended to use 5 faecal samples/ pool and to culture on solid HEY agar medium or by use of any commercial liquid culture system. Again, appropriate testing should be conducted to confirm that acid-fast isolates are *M paratuberculosis*.

1.4.5.2. Radiometric cultural method (BACTEC)

Radiometric culture techniques (BACTEC) are capable of detecting growth of Map in multiple organs including the intestinal mucosa and sub mucosa and regional lymph nodes. BACTEC culture provides a growth index of viable organisms and the number of viable organisms and this method is considered to be highly sensitive. By this technique it is possible to detect the organisms within few weeks to few days depending on the load of organisms in the samples. Some examples of this radiometric culture are BACTEC 12B and BACTEC 460. But the disadvantages of BACTEC method are, it is expensive, requires sophisticated instrumentation and it is hazardous due to complicacy of radioisotope cultures.

1.4.5.3. Agar Gel Immuno Diffusion (AGID)

Agar gel immunodiffusion (AGID) testing is used to assist in the diagnosis of clinical Johne's disease. It correlates well with heavy shedding of *M. paratuberculosis* in the faeces. But culture methods are able to detect more animals at a single test than AGID tests.

1.4.5.4. ELISA

Serum or milk samples from individual cattle can be tested by use of ELISAs. Sensitivity of ELISA for paratuberculosis is strongly dependent upon the stage of infection. Cattle that shed large numbers of organisms in their faeces and that have clinical signs compatible with paratuberculosis are most likely to have positive test results. Furthermore, a large proportion of clinically normal cattle in the early stages of infection are likely to have negative test results. This underscores the importance of repeated evaluation (bacteriologic culture of faeces and serologic testing) of cattle, coupled with management changes, to achieve effective control in herds in which paratuberculosis has been detected (Dargatz *et al.*, 2001).

1.4.5.5. Polymerase Chain Reaction (PCR)

Various mycobacteria infection can be diagnosed by PCR which provides a rapid and specific detection of Map within 24 hours to 2-3 days in some cases. Faecal samples collected from individual cattle can be tested by use of PCR assays (Wells *et al.*, 2006). Similarly, pooled faecal samples (5 faecal samples / pool) can be tested by use of PCR assays. In addition, PCR assays can be conducted on pooled faecal samples (5 faecal samples / pool) collected in accordance with Uniform Program Standards from areas in which cattle from a herd commingle. Due to presence of PCR enzyme inhibitor sometime detection of IS gene probe become difficult. Again the genetic probe based on 16s rRNA is identical for both *M. paratuberuclosis* and *M. avium* and so it could not be considered as specific probes for paratuberculosis detection. Although an improved version of immunomagnetic PCR is available for diagnosis of Map in milk samples still PCR is less sensitive than culture when applied to screen clinical samples either due to presence of inhibitory substances or non recovery of DNA. Most progress made in improving diagnosis has been made in direct detection of Map by virtue of the specific sequence IS 900 (genetic probes) and advent of gene amplification techniques like PCR. The IS900 sequence is the most commonly targeted sequence for molecular confirmation of Map, despite some concerns that the sequence may not be 100% unique to the organism.

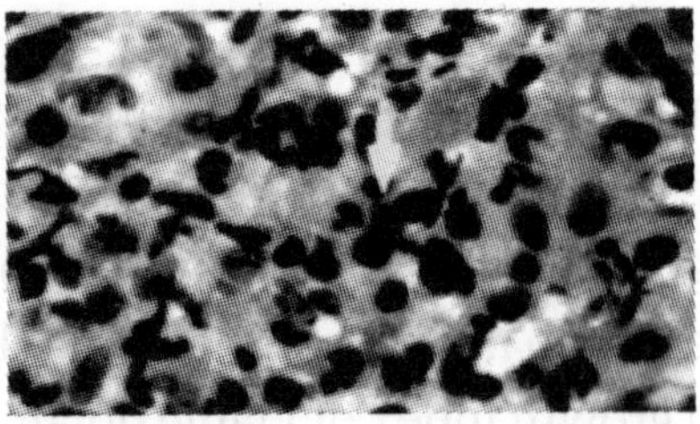

Fig. 5 : Haematoxylin and eosin staines smear of IS 900 sequence of *M. paratuberculosis*. (http://www.sciencedirect.com).

1.4.5.6. Recombinant antigen based diagnosis

In recent years recombinant antigen candidates have replaced purified antigen candidates in the development of diagnostic assays.

The advantages of recombinant antigens over purified antigens are higher product yield, high homology of antigen preparation and faster production. Several recombinant antigen candidates have been evaluated for detection of CMI against MAP.

Specificity and sensitivity of CMI based assays are poor primarily because of the applied antigens. Most studies have been conducted using PPDs (Köhler *et al.*, 2001). However, a number of studies have described novel well-defined MAP antigens for measuring CMI responses. The antigen candidates include secreted antigens, cell wall and membrane antigens, lipoproteins, heat shock proteins and hypothetical proteins. The earliest studies used native proteins purified from MAP: Avi-3 (Abe *et al.*, 1989), A36-complex (Gilot *et al.*, 1992), P30 (Burrells *et al.*, 1995), alkyl hydroperoxide reductase C (AhpC) and alkyl hydroperoxide reductase D (AhpD) (Olsen et al., 2000), MPP14 and MPB70 (Olsen *et al.*, 2005). All of these antigens were described to recall CMI responses in *in vitro* assays but they all lacked MAP specificity because of orthologues in other mycobacteria species. Two exceptions that were specific to MAP were antigens AphC and AphD, as demonstrated by immunoblot reaction of monospecific rabbit antiserum against the two antigens with 9 MAP strain lysates but not with lysates from 20 other mycobacterial species, except *M. gordonae* that produced weak cross-reactive bands (Olsen *et al.*, 2000). The diagnostic potential of AphC and AphD were evaluated in four goats experimentally infected with MAP. T cells from all four goats produced IFN-ã to *in vitro* stimulation with either antigen, whereas a non-infected control animal did not respond. AhpC and AhpD are the most promising CMI antigens among the natively purified MAP antigens as they appear to be species specific with a high sensitivity. Recently Deb and Goswami (2010 and 2011) showed that a 34.9 kDa PPE protein can be an important diagnostic against paratuberculosis.

1.4.6. Prevention and control

Control of the disease is difficult but some realistic approaches include conducting necropsy and culture examinations in large scale to get an idea of the severity of the disease in a flock, performing AGID to remove the heaviest shedders prior to calving. Testing by ELISA is recommended for control of paratuberculosis in commercial dairy herds for which the objective is to reduce economic impact of the infection. Current evidence indicates that the greatest negative economic impact is caused by cows with late-stage paratuberculosis (*i.e.*, cows with strong-positive ELISA results). is approx 85%) (Lombard *et al.*, 2005). However, when ELISAs are used, producers must act on the results in concert with risk assessment findings. Producers must be willing to cull cattle on the basis of the magnitude of an ELISA result and institute proper management of maternity pens, colostrum, and feeding of calves (Collins 1994). Analysis of data on bacterial culture of pooled faecal samples obtained from dairy cattle indicates that there is limited loss in test sensitivity and significant cost savings, compared with results for bacterial culture of individual faecal samples (Kalis *et al.*, 2000). Thus, bacterial culture of pooled faecal samples is also considered a valid testing option for eradication of paratuberculosis in a dairy herd. The best way to limit risk of purchasing infected cattle is to buy as few animals as possible. When acquisition of cattle is considered necessary, the risk is best limited through the use of tests that evaluate the infection status of the source herd rather than tests conducted on individual cattle. The situation differs among herds, partially based on the estimated infection prevalence in the buyer's herd, but the goal should be to purchase replacements from herds with a test-positive percentage that is lower than that of the buyer's herd. These recommendations are purpose-specific, scientifically sound, and economically justifiable.

1.5. Pasteurellosis with special reference to Haemorrhagic septecaemia

1.5.1. Introduction

Bovine pasteurellosis is known by a number of synonyms that are descriptive of the condition and are relevant in specific circumstances. The terms shipping fever, transit fever, bovine enzootic pneumonia, and bovine respiratory disease (BRD) complex are all very meaningful terms used to describe the disease. In the BRD complex, more than one species and serotype of pasteurellae are incriminated as playing a role that is secondary to respiratory viruses and 'stress'. However, Haemorrhagic septicaemia (HS) is a primary pasteurellosis caused by specific serotypes of the species *P. multocida*. In India, HS accounted for 46–55% of all bovine deaths. During the twelve years period since 1974 to 1986 it accounted for 58.7% of the aggregate of deaths due to five endemic diseases *viz.*, foot-and-mouth disease (FMD), rinderpest, blackquarter, anthrax and HS (Dutta *et al.*, 1990).

1.5.2. Etiological agents

H.S is caused by *Pasteurella multocida*, a Gram-negative coccobacillus residing mostly as a commensal in the upper respiratory tract of animals. The Asian serotype B:2 and the African serotype E:2 (Carter and Heddleston system), corresponding to 6:B and 6:E (Namioka-carter system), are mainly responsible for the disease. In wild animals, serotype B:2,5 are predominantly present. The association of other serotypes, namely A:1, A:3 with a HS-like condition in cattle in India has been recorded (Kumar *et al.*, 1996). The pasteurellae associated with BRD are predominantly *P. haemolytica* type A, and *P. multocida* capsular serogroup A. There is no consistency in the somatic types involved. The pasteurellae that cause pneumonic pasteurellosis are carried in the upper respiratory tract (URT) of *calves.* In the case of *P. haemolytica* type A 1, the bacterium is not easily detected in the URT of healthy calves, but is shed and can be easily isolated in calves that are stressed in some way or affected with another concurrent infection. The URTs of stressed or otherwise diseased calves can be easily colonised by *P. haemolytica* A 1. In the case of *P. multocida,* no such relationship between stress and ability to colonise has been observed. The organism causing HS does not survive outside the animal body to any significant degree so as to be a source of infection. Moist conditions prolong its survival. Thus, the disease tends to spread more during the wet season (De Alwis 1990a).

Table 1 : Diseases caused by *Pasteurella* organisms in cattle in India

Disease	Organism(s)
Haemorrhagic septicaemia	*P. multocida* serotype B:2 and E:2
H.S like septicaemic disease	*P. multocida* serotype B: 3,4
Bovine pneumonic pasteurellosis	*P. haemolytica* A1 and *P. mutocida* A

1.5.3. Epidemiology of H.S

Hemorrhagic septicemia in epidemic form is a disease mainly of cattle and water buffaloes either maintained separately or together. Radical changes in weather, including the advent of monsoons, debility caused by seasonal levels of low nutrition, and the pressure of work as it occurs in case of draft animals are related to the explosive occurrences of the disease in certain parts of the world. Southeast Asia, where such conditions often coincide, is the area of highest incidence. The disease occurs in the Middle East and Africa where the environmental circumstances and predisposing conditions are not as clearly defined as in Southeast Asia. As in India, the disease is frequently associated with the rainy season and poor physical condition.

The disease is spread by either direct or indirect contact via fomites. The source of the infection is infected animals or carriers. The carrier state may be greater than 20 percent shortly after an outbreak, but within 6 weeks the rate is usually less than 5 percent. The causal agent does not survive for more than 2 to 3 weeks in the soil or on pastures. Close herding and wetness, as occurs during the rainy season, appear to contribute to spread. There is no evidence that biting arthropods are significant vectors. The extrinsic factors have direct influence in the development of the clinical pasteurelloses, and particularly in hemorrhagic septicaemia. When favorable circumstances for the growth and multiplication of *P. multocida* in the animal body occur, severe septicemia develops within a few hours. However, the organisms may be harbored for varying periods in a small percentage of carrier animals without any clinical sign. The perpetuation of the disease from year to year or season to season is generally attributed to the carrier state. The immune status of the animal is thought to influence the severity of the disease.

1.5.4. Clinical signs and post mortem lesions

The majority of cases in cattle are acute or per acute with death occurring from 6 to 24 hours after the first recognized signs. In a few outbreaks, animals may survive as long as 72 hours. The first signs are dullness, reluctance to move, and elevated temperature. Following these signs, salivation and nasal discharge appear, and oedematous swellings are seen in the pharyngeal region and then spread to the ventral cervical region and brisket. Visible mucous membranes are congested, and respiratory distress is soon followed by collapse and death. Recovery is rare. Chronic manifestations of hemorrhagic septicaemia do not appear to occur. Husbandry, weather and immunity affect morbidity. In endemic areas, 10 to 50 percent of the cattle population acquire solid immunity through exposure or subclinical infection. Close herding and wetness predispose to an increased morbidity. Most animals that develop clinical sign die.

Widely distributed hemorrhages, oedema and general hyperemia are the most obvious tissue changes observed in infected animals at necropsy. In almost all cases there is an oedematous swelling of the head, neck and brisket region. Incision of the oedematous swellings reveals a coagulated sero-fibrinous mass with straw colored or blood-stained fluid. This type of oedema that distends tissue spaces is also found in the musculature. Subserosal petechial hemorrhages are also found throughout the carcass, and blood-tinged fluid is frequently found in the thoracic and abdominal cavities. Pharyngeal and cervical lymph nodes are found to be swollen, haemorrhagic and petechiae may be observed. However, pneumonia and gastroenteritis are not observed frequently.

1.5.5. Diagnosis

1.5.5.1. Differential diagnosis

The disease should be differentiated from other causes of sudden death such as lightning strikes, blackleg (*Clostridium chauveoi* infection), rinderpest and anthrax. Acute salmonellosis and pneumonic pasteurellosis should also be taken into consideration.

1.5.5.2. Cultural and biochemical identification

Isolation is more likely to be successful if a fresh sample that is free from contaminating bacteria and post–mortem invaders can be collected. In Gram–stained blood or tissue smears, *P. multocida* is a Gram–negative, short bacillus or ovoid form with bipolar staining. Bipolar staining is more apparent with methylene blue or Leishman's stain, and may be lost after serial passage. Some pleomorphism can be expected, especially in older cultures. *P. multocida* can be grown on blood agar, chocolate agar or casein/sucrose/yeast (CSY) agar with 5% blood. Dextrose starch agar or trypticase soya agar may also be used. Freshly isolated *P. multocida* colonies are smooth, nonhemolytic, grayish, translucent, glistening and approximately 1 mm in diameter after incubation on blood agar for 24 hours at 37°C. Larger colonies are seen on CSY agar, and smaller colonies may develop from old cultures.

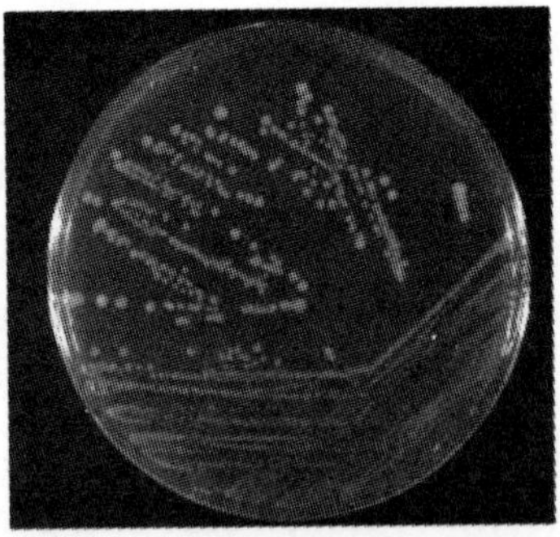

Fig. 6 : Non-haemolytic colonies of *P. multocida* on Blood agar http://www.ehs.uc.edu.

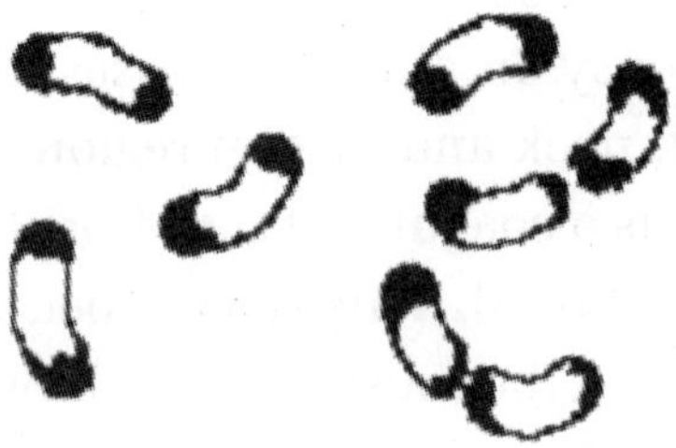

Fig. 7 : Bipolar staining property of *P. multocida* (http://www.library. tcmedc.org)

One property of HS-causing strains of *P. multocida* is the ability to produce the enzyme hyaluronidase (Carter and Chengappa 1980). Hyaluronidase production can be used as a specific test for HS-causing pasteurellae after identifying the genus and species by cultural characters. However, that B serotypes other than B:2 (or 6:B) and type E are hyaluronidase negative.

1.5.5.3. Tests for serotyping

Tests used for serotyping include a rapid slide agglutination test or indirect hemagglutination test for capsular typing, an agglutination test for somatic typing, agar gel immunodiffusion for both capsular and somatic typing and counter-immunoelectrophoresis for the rapid identification of the capsular types B and E. Broadly, two typing systems are adopted. One is 'capsular' typing by Carter's Indirect Haemagglutination (IHA) test or by AGID tests. The other is somatic typing by the method of Namioka & Murata, and by the method of Heddleston. It is generally agreed that designation of serotypes should be based on a somatic– capsular combination. Two systems commonly in use are the Namioka–Carter and the Carter–Heddleston systems. In the former system, Asian and African HS serotypes are designated 6:B and 6:E, respectively, while in the latter system they are designated B.2 and E.2, respectively.

1.5.5.4. Nucleic acid recognition methods

Polymerase chain reaction (PCR) techniques can detect organisms in clinical samples and bacterial cultures. *P. multocida* multiplex capsular PCR typing system can be used for identification of the genes involved in the biosynthesis of the *P. multocida* A:1 (20) and B:2 polysaccharide capsules provided the required information to determine the biosynthetic region of the remaining three serogroups *viz.*, D, E, and F (Boyce *et al.*, 2000). Moreover, with the use of serogroup specific multiplex PCR, conflicting results in relation to typing of some strains can be confirmed. Presumptive identification of HS-causing type-B-specific *P. multocida* is also possible by PCR amplification. Comparative analysis with the *Haemophilus influenzae* Rd genome indicates that DNA regions amplified in both assays reside in close proximity, yet slight differences in specificity are evident. The HS-causing type-B-specific PCR remains 100% specific for HS-causing type B serotypes of isolated *P. multocida* (Townsend *et al.*, 1998). DNA fingerprinting and other genetic methods can characterize isolates further for epidemiological investigations, but are generally available only in research laboratories.

1.5.6. Prevention and control

Vaccination is a major control measure in the face of a new epidemic. Various vaccine types have been developed *viz.*, the broth bacterin, the oil adjuvant vaccine, the double emulsion vaccine and a live vaccine (Verma and Jaiswal, 1998). During an outbreak, one should resort to immediate whole herd vaccination, irrespective of previous vaccination history. The use of either broth bacterin or oil adjuvant vaccine is recommended. Sanitary measures include early detection and isolation of new cases and their immediate treatment with antibiotics, deep burial of carcasses or incineration, and the prevention of movements of animals to disease free areas.

Import of animals from an area of unknown status to a free area should comply with some practical procedures which should take into account the high percentage of carriers that occur in endemic areas than was earlier believed, and the persistence of the carrier status for long periods (De Alwis *et al.*, 1990b). Briefly, these include ensuring the origin of the animals from a region where no outbreaks of HS have occurred for a minimum period of one year, carrying out an indirect haemagglutination (IHA) testing on the animals to be exported, holding animals under observation for 2–3 weeks before transport, quarantining them for the same period of time upon arrival to destination and to vaccinate all animals at the end of the quarantine period. Whenever animals are exported from HS endemic countries, even after observing all the above precautions, it is important to vaccinate all susceptible stock in the importing area that are likely to come into contact with the imported animals.

1.6. Leptospirosis

1.6.1. Introduction

Leptospirosis is an economically important zoonotic bacterial infection of livestock that causes abortions, stillbirths, infertility and loss of milk production. The disease occurs worldwide and is caused by infection with the spirochete Leptospira. It is an infectious and contagious bacterial disease of most farm animals and many wildlife species. In cattle, leptospirosis can produce an abortion rate of up to 30 per cent when it occurs during the final third of pregnancy. It may also be responsible for high mortality among young calves, decreased milk production, and blood-contaminated milk. Severity in adult cattle is extremely variable, ranging from inapparent infection to 5 percent mortality. The causative organisms, called Leptospires, are shed in urine and survive in surface water, streams, or moist, alkaline soil.

1.6.2. Etiological agent

The pathogenic leptospires were formerly classified as members of the species Leptospira interrogans; the genus has recently been reorganized and pathogenic leptospires are now identified in 7 species of Leptospira. Approximately 200 different serovars of pathogenic Leptospira have been identified throughout the world. Serovars are identified based on antigens on the surface of the organisms. Some examples of different serovars include *hardjo, pomona, canicola, icterohaemorrhagiae,* and *grippotyphosa* (Bolin 2003). The most common cause of leptospirosis among cattle throughout much of the world is infection with leptospires belonging to serovar Hardjo. Two serologically indistinguishable but genetically distinct types of serovar Hardjo have been identified: *Leptospira interrogans* serovar *Hardjo* (type hardjoprajitno) and *L. borgpetersenii* serovar *Hardjo* (type *hardjo-bovis*). Serovar Hardjo type hardjo-bovis is common in cattle populations throughout the world including India.

1.6.3. Epidemiology

Serovars are typically associated with one or more maintenance hosts that serve as reservoirs of infection. Maintenance hosts can be wildlife species or domestic animals, including livestock. An animal may be infected by serovars maintained by its own species which is called maintenance host infection / host-adapted infection or serovars maintained by other species which is called incidental infection / nonhost-adapted infection (www.aces.edu).

Table 2 : *Leptospira* serovars and their maintenance hosts

***Leptospira* serovars**	**Maintenace hosts**
Hardjo—bovis	Cattle
Pomona	Pigs, skunks
Canicola	Dogs
Icterohaemorrhagiae	Rats, other rodents
Grippotyphosa	Raccoons, skunks, opposums
Bratislava	Pigs, horses

Leptospira hardjo-bovis is the only host-adapted Lepto serovar in cattle and can infect animals at any age, including young calves. Because cattle are the maintenance host for *hardjo-bovis*, infection with this serovar will often produce a carrier state in the kidneys associated with long-term urinary shedding. In addition, infections with *hardjo-bovis* can persist in the reproductive tract.

The disease is transmitted either directly between animals or indirectly through the environment. The *Leptospira* organism is most commonly shed in the urine of an infected animal and can even be shed through aborted fetuses, thus infecting animals directly or contaminating the environment. The source of infection can therefore be an infected animal or water/feed that has been contaminated with infected urine. The organisms gain entry to the body though the membranes of the eyes, nose, mouth, and even the skin, especially if it is injured or water softened. Infected animals also commonly shed the bacteria in placental fluids and milk. In addition, some *Leptospira* serovars can be transmitted venereally through sexual contact.

The organisms can survive in the environment for weeks to months depending on environmental conditions and some organisms can survive in stagnant, standing water or in wet soil for longer than six months if the temperature is favourable and ranges between 50° and 93° F. Moisture and warm temperatures are conducive to *Leptospira* survival, while dry, freezing, and extremely high temperatures often kill the bacteria.

1.6.4. Clinical signs

Infection by serovar *Hardjo* generally results in relatively mild acute clinical signs but produces a renal carrier state associated with long-term urinary shedding. Persistent infection of the male and female genital tract is also a prominent feature of serovar *Hardjo* infections. Clinical signs of serovar *Hardjo* infection in dairy cattle are mild and generally involve decreased reproductive efficiency and milk production. Abortions, stillbirths, or birth of weak calves occur as a result of serovar *Hardjo* infection but generally, are only seen when a cow is infected for the first time when she is pregnant. Abortions may occur many weeks after infection of the dam and are usually not associated with any obvious illness in the cow. Infected, but apparently healthy, calves also may be born and retention of fetal membranes may follow *Hardjo* abortion. In contrast to abortion storms caused by serovars *Pomona* and *Grippotyphosa*, abortion due to serovar *Hardjo* tend to occur sporadically.

1.6.5. Diagnosis

Diagnosis of leptospirosis is dependant on a good clinical and vaccination history and the availability of diagnostic testing at a laboratory with experience in the diagnosis of leptospirosis. The tests can be separated into those designed to detect antibodies against the organism and those designed to detect the organism or its' DNA in tissues or body fluids of animals. Each of the diagnostic procedures, for detection of the organism or for antibodies directed against the organisms, has a number of advantages and disadvantages. Some of the assays suffer from a lack of sensitivity and others are prone to specificity problems. Therefore, no single technique can be recommended for use in each clinical situation. Use of a combination of tests allows maximum sensitivity and specificity in establishing the diagnosis.

1.6.5.1. Cultural examination

The organism may be identified by dark field examination of blood or by culture on a semisolid medium like Fletcher's EMJH *i.e.* Ellinghausen-McCullough-Johnson- Harris if taken before the tenth day of illness. Cultures take 1-6 weeks to become positive. The organism can also be isolated from the urine on darkground microscopy tenth day onwards.

1.6.5.2. Serological tests

1.6.5.2.1. Microscopic agglutination test (MAT)

The microscopic agglutination test (MAT) is the most commonly used technique for diagnosing leptospirosis in animals. Serology is inexpensive, reasonably sensitive, and widely available. The MAT involves mixing appropriate dilutions of serum with live leptospires of serovars prevalent within the region. The presence of antibodies is indicated by the agglutination of the leptospires. Detection of high titers of antibody in animals with a disease consistent with leptospirosis may be sufficient to establish the diagnosis. This is particularly true in the investigation of abortions caused by incidental host infections in which the dam's agglutinating antibody titer is greater than 1:800-1600. Interpretation of leptospiral serologic results is complicated by a number of factors *viz.*, cross-reactivity of antibodies, antibody titers induced by vaccination, and lack of consensus about what antibody titers are indicative of active infection.

1.6.5.2.2. Recombinant antigen based ELISA

Recombinant antigen based single serum dilution ELISA makes use of the recombinant LipL32 antigen developed from the serovar *Pomona* strain *Pomona* of the pathogenic *L. interrogans* species. The r LipL32 ELISA has been found to be sensitive, specific and accurate as compared to the standard MAT and the test can be efficiently utilized as a screening test for a large number of human serum samples for the detection of leptospiral antibodies (Dey *et al.*, 2008).

1.6.5.3. Detection of Leptospires

1.6.5.3.1. Immunofluorescence

Immunofluorescence can be used to identify leptospires in tissues, blood, or urine sediment. The availability of this test is increasing, and the test is rapid, has good sensitivity, and is very useful for screening urine samples or fetal tissues for leptospires. Interpretation of immunofluorescence tests may be difficult and some diagnostic labs may be more experienced with this test than others. The fluorescent antibody conjugate currently in general use is not serovar-specific. Serologic examination of the animal is still required to identify the infecting serovar (Faine 1982).

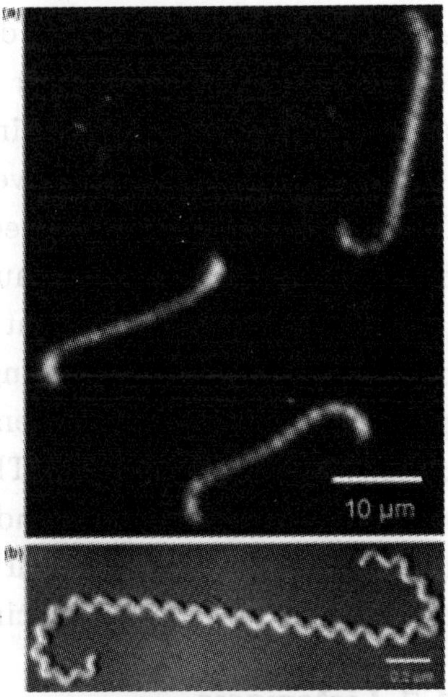

Fig. 8 : Dark field (a) Shadowed electron and (b) Photomicrographs of *Leptospira* spp. http://www.sciencedirect.com.

1.6.5.3.2. PCR

PCR methods appear to be sensitive, specific, positive early in disease, and able to detect leptospiral DNA in blood, urine, cerebrospinal fluid (CSF) and aqueous humor. A number of PCR procedures are available and each laboratory running the test may select a slightly different procedure that works well for them. In general, PCR testing of urine is more reliable than testing of tissues. But major disadvantage with these tests is that these are genus-specific, not serovar specific (Dutta and Christopher 2005).

1.6.6. Prevention and control

Because of the presence of *Leptospira* carrier states in both cattle and wildlife, avoiding all exposure to leptospirosis is not possible for most beef cattle operations. Infected bulls, of course, should never be used for natural service or artificial insemination until they have been treated to eliminate shedding and are subsequently tested, examined, and found free of disease. However, attempting to prevent leptospirosis through regular herd vaccination is the best approach. At a minimum, annual vaccination of bulls, cows, and replacement heifers at least six to eight weeks before the breeding season with a five-way Lepto vaccine is recommended after initial primary and booster vaccinations. Because all Lepto vaccines are killed, or inactivated, it is essential that animals receive the initial primary and booster vaccinations according to label directions, which include the proper time interval between the initial and booster vaccinations, usually about four weeks. The vaccination of animals less than 3 months old is not recommended due to possible residual antibodies, but vaccination of cows in early to mid-pregnancy use to protect their calves. The best time to vaccinate cows is 30 days before breeding.

1.7. Listeriosis

1.7.1. Introduction

A wide variety of animal species can be infected with *Listeria monocytogenes*, but clinical listeriosis is mainly a ruminant disease including cattle, with occasional sporadic cases in other species. The main clinical manifestations of animal listeriosis are encephalitis, septicaemia, abortion and the disease is often associated with stored forages, usually silage. Most infections in animals are subclinical, but listeriosis can occur either sporadically or in epidemic form. In addition to the economic impact of listeriosis in animals, there is a link between animals and their role as a source of infection for humans primarily from consumption of contaminated animal products.

1.7.2. Etiological agent

Listeria monocytogenes (Lm) which is a normal saprophyte of the soil, contaminated water and spoiled, concentrated hay or silage. It can live in soil and faecal contents for a long time.

1.7.3. Epidemiology

The organism is transmitted from animal to animal through fecal oral routes, usually via manure contamination of the pasture or silage with the micro organism. Animal to human transmission is either directly through direct contact with infected animals or indirectly via milk, cheese, meat, eggs, or vegetables (Wesley 1999). After infecting, the bacteria multiply and spread throughout the animal's body causing fever and decreased appetite. Listeriosis affects all ages and sexes, but animals less than three years of age are more commonly prone to clinical disease.

1.7.4. Clinical signs and post mortem findings

The clinical manifestations of listeriosis in animals include encephalitis, septicaemia and abortion in cattle. The septicaemic form is relatively uncommon and generally occurs in the neonate. It is characterized by depression, inappetence, fever and death. The encephalitic form is sometimes referred to as 'circling disease' because of a tendency to circle in one direction, and it is the most common manifestation of the disease in ruminants. The signs include depression, anorexia, head pressing or turning of the head to one side and unilateral facial paralysis. Abortion usually occurs after 7 months. Only one clinical form of listeriosis usually occurs in a particular group of animals. Bovine ophthalmitis have also been described (Walker 1999). Rarely *L. monocytogenes* infection is associated with mastitis.

The post-mortem findings and histopathology depend on the clinical presentation. In the encephalitic form, the cerebrospinal fluid may be cloudy and the meningeal vessels congested. Gross pathological lesions of the brain are rare. On occasion, the medulla shows areas of softening. However, the histopathology is characteristic of the disease, consisting of foci of inflammatory cells with adjacent perivascular cuffing, predominantly of lymphocytes and histiocytes, plasma cells and occasional neutrophils. The microabscesses in the brain stem severely affect one side of the brain. In the septicaemic form, multiple foci of necrosis in the liver and, less frequently the spleen, may be noted. Aborted fetuses of ruminants show very little gross lesions, but autolysis may be present if the fetus is retained before expulsion (Low and Donachie 1997).

1.7.5. Diagnosis

A definitive diagnosis can only be made at postmortem by histopathology of the pontomedullary region of the brainstem and by bacterial culture. Usually there are no gross lesions seen in the brain at necropsy. The characteristic microscopic lesions include multifocal asymmetrical microabscesses and mononuclear cell meningoencephalitis in the brainstem, anterior spinal cord and, occasionally, cerebellum. The motility of the organism can be demonsrated by hanging drop technique in wet mount preparation. Peroxidase-antiperoxidase test, a more accurate diagnostic tool than histopathology, is used to detect degraded bacterial proteins as well as intact bacteria in formalin-fixed tissue.

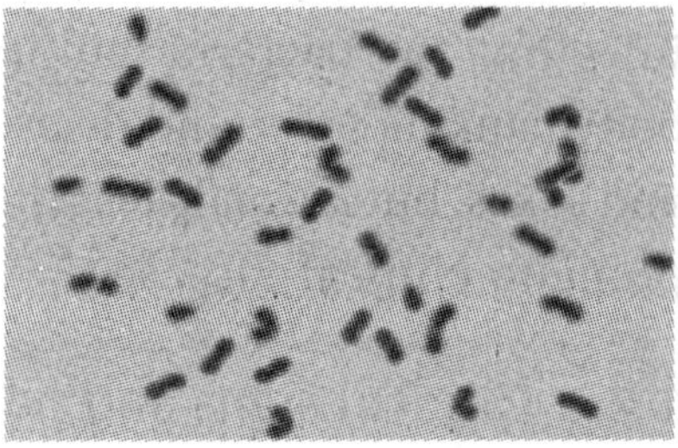

Fig. 9 : *L. monocytogenes* demonstrated by wet mount technique. http://www.811699.net.

1.7.5.1. Cultural examination

Bacteriological diagnosis of animal listeriosis has traditionally involved direct plating of specimens on blood agar or other enriched media and concomitant use of the 'cold enrichment' technique, with weekly subculturing for up to 12 weeks (Quinn *et al.*, 1999). Immunohistochemical detection of *L. monocytogenes* antigens in formalin-fixed tissue has proven to be more sensitive than direct plating and cold enrichment bacterial culture for the diagnosis of the encephalitic form of the disease in ruminants (Campero *et al.*, 2002). The introduction of alternative enrichment procedures and selective agents for the isolation of *L. monocytogenes* from food and environmental samples has opened up the possibility of using some of these techniques for the bacteriological analysis of samples.

1.7.5.2. Rapid serological and molecular identification

1.7.5.2.1. Colorimetric monoclonal enzyme-linked immunosorbent assay

It is intended for the detection of *Listeria* spp. in dairy products, seafood and meats. The test is not confirmatory for *L. monocytogenes* as the monoclonal antibodies (MAbs) used in the test may cross react with other *Listeria* spp. Enrichment cultures found positive by this method are streaked on selective media and suspect colonies are biochemically identified as *L. monocytogenes* according to the FDA method. A positive result is only valid when the positive and negative controls give acceptable absorbance readings (AOAC 2000).

1.7.5.2.2. Polymerase chain reaction

Polymerase chain reaction (PCR), targeting the *hly* gene, has been found to be a sensitive and rapid technique for confirmation of the identification of suspect *L. monocytogenes* isolated on selective/ differential agar plates (Gouws and Liedemann 2005).

1.7.5.3. Subtyping methods

Strains of *Listeria* can be assigned to 13 different serotypes, based on their combination of somatic (O) and flagellar (H) antigens. Bacteriophage typing is a technique with very good discriminatory power that can be used to subtype a large number of isolates. However, the current available phage sets are unable to type a high proportion of strains. However, inspite of this problem, phage typing remains the most practical and suitable method for application in large acute outbreaks (Graves *et al.*, 1999). Although there have been some reports on the sequence analysis of single genes as a means to type *L. monocytogenes* strains, determination of allelic variation of multiple genes by multi locus sequence typing (MLST) has been recently introduced as a very promising subtyping methodology for this microorganism. Direct amplification and nucleotide sequencing (Salcedo *et al.*, 2003), as well as an alternative approach that targets the variable genetic changes directly in a DNA array format (Rudi *et al.*, 2003) have both been used with good discrimination between the strains analysed. As MLST is based on nucleotide sequence, it is highly discriminatory and provides unambiguous results.

1.7.6. Prevention and control

Prevention is the key to listeriosis. In the livestock industry, feeding of spoiled silage and other rotten vegetation should be avoided and sick animals should be isolated from the healthy animals. There is a well-established linkage between silage feeding and listeriosis and, as *L. monocytogenes* is widely distributed in nature, with animals and birds acting as carriers, contamination of silage is not uncommon. Emphasis should therefore be placed on reducing the likelihood of the multiplication of the organism, which occurs more frequently at pH values greater than 5, particularly where ineffective fermentation has occurred and where there is concomitant growth of moulds. Every effort should be made to produce silage of good quality, with early cutting of grass, minimal contamination with soil or faeces and ensuring optimal anaerobic fermentation, which will insure that the pH falls below 5.0 and at that level, growth of *Listeria* spp. is inhibited (OIE 2008). Good hygiene and sanitation on the farm is also important. Whenever possible, people at risk for listeriosis should avoid the consumption of foods associated with listeriosis. Livestock and crop producers can also help to control the spread of *L. monocytogenes* by avoiding the use of untreated manure on vegetable crops.

To develop effective vaccines against *L. monocytogenes* is found to be very difficult as it is an intracellular organism and requires effector T cells for an effective immune response. Experimental vaccines in laboratory animals are being explored to confer protection to *L. monocytogenes* infection by a number of different approaches, but these are still far from becoming available for human and farm animal use. These experimental approaches include immunisation with plasmid DNA, CD40 signalling along with heat-killed *L. monocytogenes*, LLO-deficient mutants inoculated along with liposome-encapsulated LLO, and immunisation with listerial antigens and IL-12. Genetically modified *L. monocytogenes* is also being considered as an effective vaccine vector for the expression, secretion and intracellular delivery of foreign antigens for the induction of potent immune responses against viral antigens and tumour cells.

1.8. Clostridial infections

1.8.1. Introduction

Clostridial diseases are caused by bacteria of the genus *Clostridium*. Clostridia are widespread in the environment and are normally found in soil and faeces. They form highly resistant spores that can survive in the environment for very long periods. They are also present in the gastrointestinal tract and as spores in tissues of healthy animals (Robson 2007). Not all species of clostridia cause disease, but those that do are usually fatal. Disease occurs when these bacteria enter the body via cuts, abrasions or ingestion and conditions in the body allow multiplication of the bacteria and toxin production. Clostridial diseases are typically infectious but not contagious. In other words, cattle that become infected will not directly transmit the disease to other cattle. Animals afflicted with clostridial diseases usually die very quickly, sometimes without any prior clinical signs. Therefore, prevention of these diseases through the use of vaccines is often much more successful than trying to treat infected animals.

1.8.2. Etiological agent

Clostridial bacteria produce long-lived structures called endospores. Endospores are forms of bacteria that are extremely resistant to environmental conditions *viz.*, heat, drought, UV radiation and chemical disinfectants. When endospores are introduced into an animal, they can develop into the infectious bacteria. Once the bacteria begin to grow, they cause disease by producing and releasing toxins into the calf's body.

Table 3 : Diseases caused by different Clostridial spp.

Clostridium	Diseases caused
C. tetani	Tetanus
C. septicum	Malignant oedema
C. chauvoei	Black quarter
C. perfringens	Abomasitis,haemorrhagic enteritis,Enterotoxaemia (Pulpy kidney)
C. novyi	Black disease
C. botulinum	Botulism

1.8.3. Tetanus

Tetanus usually results from contamination of deep puncture wounds. Castration and dehorning wounds are another risk, as are wounds from calving trauma. *Clostridium tetani* organisms remain at the site of entry, multiply, and produce a toxin that affects the nervous system, causing stimulation and contraction of the skeletal muscles. The incubation period for tetanus is approximately 10 to 21 days. The affected animal will appear stiff, the tail is held out, the head and neck stretched out, the third eyelid comes across the eye and the nostrils are flared. Bloat is common. As the disease progresses, a 'sawhorse' stance is adopted, and 'lockjaw' develops. Eventually the animal will not be able to stand and goes into 'tetanic' convulsions. Respiratory failure ends in death. Tetanus can be treated with penicillin, tetanus antitoxin and supportive therapy. Tranquilizers may need to be administered to control seizures. Intravenous fluids are indicated to control dehydration if the animal cannot eat or drink. Prevention can be achieved through the use of vaccination injections and being diligent about using clean instruments when performing invasive procedures (Smith 1996). Immunity can be provided by antitoxin. Dose of homologous antitoxin is 400IU in animals and 40 IU in human. Toxoids are of value in preventing tetanus. Vaccination is done when the kids are about 10 weeks of age. At this time their immune systems are mature enough to provide lasting immunity. Maternal antibodies through colostrums provides lasting immunity maximum upto 12 weeks.

1.8.4. Malignant oedema

Clostridium septicum is the agent causing malignant edema. Malignant edema is generally fatal in cattle and can affect cattle of any age. *Clostridium septicum* is found in the intestinal tracts of most domestic livestock, and it is shed in their faeces, leading to pasture contamination. This disease develops when an open wound caused by accidental injury, castration or difficult parturition gets infected with the bacteria. Infection can also occur via the umbilicus in newborn calves and following injections if proper aseptic technique is not used. Toxins are produced at the entry site. This causes extensive swelling, with accumulation of bloody or clear fluid, and tissue death followed by gangrene. The affected area is extremely painful. Toxins are absorbed into the bloodstream, causing fever, weakness, trembling, and then death. Lesions in the dead animal include darkened discoloration of the affected tissue and a foul odour and soft tissue swelling without gas accumulation will be associated with the diseased tissue. Treatment with penicillin is only effective if started very early in the disease onset as the course of the disease leading to death is very rapid. Vaccination is the most reliable form of control.

1.8.5. Black quarter

Black quarter also known as blackleg affects cattle worldwide and is caused by *Clostridium chauvoei* and begins when the susceptible animal ingests the endospores. The endospores then cross over the gastrointestinal tract and enter the bloodstream. Endospores are deposited in tissue throughout the animal's body. They lie dormant in the tissue until they become activated and trigger the disease. This bacterium is activated in an oxygen deficient environment and hence requires a site where there is low oxygen content, such as damaged, devitalized or bruised tissue. The damaged muscle tissue will have a compromised blood flow as a result of which oxygen will not be as readily delivered to the affected area. Therefore, any activity that causes bruising can promote the disease. Once this stimulating event occurs, the spores germinate and multiply into the disease-causing bacteria. Disease can develop without any history of wounds to the animal.

Although blackleg has occurred in calves as young as 2 months of age, the disease generally affects animals between 6 months and 2 years of age. Occasionally, losses may be seen in adult cattle. Blackleg infections typically occur during the late summer and early fall and affects rapidly growing calves. It may be noted in flooded areas which allows the spores to rise to the surface of the ground. It may also occur during times of drought when the grass is very low, and cattle will ingest spores from the soil during grazing.

Typically, animals infected with blackleg die rapidly without any signs of illness. However, clinical signs that may be noted very early in the disease include lameness, loss of appetite, fever and depression. Animals quickly die within 12 to 48 hours after contracting the disease. Although treatment usually fails, appropriate doses of penicillin may prove helpful. If an animal does survive, it will likely suffer from a permanent deformity. Lesions in a dead animal associated with blackleg include swelling of the affected muscle tissue of legs, neck, hip, chest, shoulder or back. The swelling is due to fluid and gas accumulation which is produced by the infectious bacteria. When pressure is applied to the affected areas, gas can often be felt moving while producing a crackling sound under the skin. Affected muscle tissue contains dark areas of necrotic tissue and may also have a foul odor which is usually described as rancid butter. Gangrenous changes may even occur in the heart muscle.

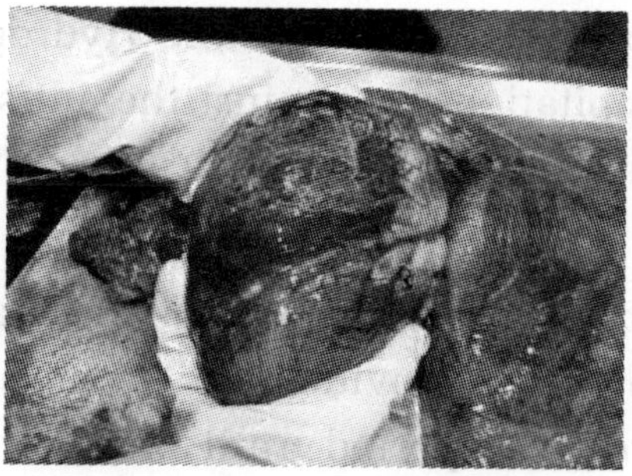

Fig. 10 : Gangrenous changes in heart muscle affected by *Cl. chouvei* http://www.sdstate.edu.

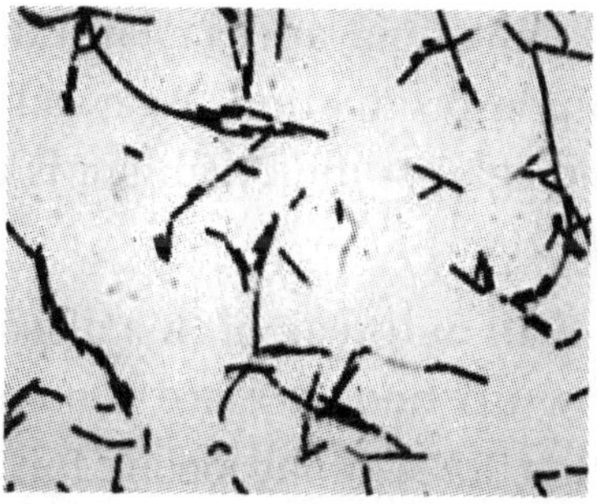

Fig. 11 : *Cl. chouvei* in tissue smear stained by gram's staining technique http://vet.uga.edu.

The isolation of *C. chauvoei* from muscle lesion is problematic because of the rapidity with which other *Clostridia* invade the tissues from the gastro-intestinal tract after death and the fastidiousness of the organism in the culure (Williams 1977). Isolations are thus made only from affected muscles not showing the visible evidence of putrifaction and decomposition. Suspensions made from muscle sample when inoculated without calcium chloride solution causes no death in guineapig. However, when these suspensions are inoculated with 3 per cent calcium chloride solution causes death in guineapigs within 24 to 72 hours of inoculation as calcium chloride not only activates the spores but also helps in germination of spores by damaging the local tissues and thereby producing anaerobiasis (Princewell 1965). The heart blood, liver and thigh muscles from dead guineapigs can be cultured on freshly poured blood agar plates, bullock heart medium and Tarozzi medium. On blood agar, organisms produce 2 to 3 mm diameter colonies which are slightly raised and whitish grey in colour with glossy surface and the entire margin surrounded by narrow zone of haemolysis. Organisms produce turbidity and large amount of gas in bullock heart medium and Tarozzi medium. Microscopically, the isolates appear gram-positive, short rods with rounded ends, occurring singly or in short chains of 2-5 organisms with oval shaped spores wider than the cell giving it a pear shaped appearance. Biochemically, the organisms utilize lactose and sucrose producing acid and gas and are positive for catalase and Hydrogen sulphide production. Agar gel precipitation test against the antisera raised against the organism is a remarkable immunological test (Naz *et al.*, 2005).

If an outbreak of this disease occurs, immediate vaccination and follow-up boosters are recommended to provide good immunity. Further losses may occur for a two-week period until the animals develop ample immunity against the disease. Carcass disposal should be done carefully after an outbreak of disease occurs. If possible carcasses should be buries deeply where they lie. Dragging of carcasses across the pastures should be avoided as it can contaminate the ground more.

1.8.6. Infections caused by *C. perfringens*

There are five types of *C. perfringens* designated as A to E, which are identified based on the toxins they produce. It is the effect of these specific toxins that results in the clinical signs and syndrome attributable to each type.

Table 4 : ***Clostridium perfringens*** **types, major toxins and associated syndromes**

Type	Major toxin	Associated syndrome
A	Alpha	Abomasitis, bloating and haemorrhagic bowel syndrome in calves
B	Alpha, Beta, Epsilon	Haemorrhagic enteritis in new borne calves
C	Alpha, Beta	Bloody scour
D	Alpha, Epsilon	Enterotoxaemia in finishing cattle
E	Alpha, Iota	Fatal enterotoxaemia in new borne calves

Clostridium perfringens Type A has been increasingly identified as a cause of abomasal inflammation, which may result in abdominal distension / bloating and abomasal ulcers in young calves. Varying degrees of diarrhea and sudden onset of weakness and coma have also been associated with Type A which generally affects 2-4 weeks old calf. It is also occasionally associated with wound contamination and gas gangrene. Type B is almost non-existent. Type C is one of the more commonly encountered types of C. perfringens. It is especially virulent in calves less than 10 days old and often less than 5 days old. Enterotoxemia due to *C. perfringens* Type C may result in severe bloody diarrhea but calves may die before the onset of diarrhea. Enterotoxemia due to *C. perfringens* Type D is sometimes associated with sudden death in finishing cattle because it proliferates when there are high amounts of carbohydrates available in the diet, which is often the case in cattle being fed high amounts of grain in finishing diets. A number of toxins are produced, but the most important toxin damages blood vessels and the nervous system. The disease also tends to occur in young, rapidly growing animals in good condition and on a high plane of nutrition. A disruption in digestion is necessary for the disease to occur. Type E enterotoxemia is responsible for a severe local intestinal necrosis and systemic toxemia similar to the syndrome described with Type C (Daly 2007).

Necropsy of the calf, in cases of Types C and E sometimes reveal severe necrosis and hemorrhage in the small intestine. Calves affected with Type A often show inflammation, ulceration, and hemorrhage of the lining of the rumen and abomasum. As *C. perfringens* is often found in the intestine of normal calves, a simple culture of the organism from the calf is not sufficient by itself to confirm a diagnosis of disease. Culture results are matched with clinical signs, lesions in the tissues, and, in some cases, toxin identification, to obtain a true diagnosis. Tissue samples from calves suspected of having clostridial enterotoxemia should be collected soon after death and kept well-preserved.

Despite the fact that clostridial organisms are ubiquitous in the calf's environment, the more organisms a newborn calf is exposed to, the more likely it is to succumb to the disease. Hence, careful attention must be paid to sanitation of the calving area. Buildup of all enteric pathogens occurs when the same calving area is used throughout the calving season as these organisms are generally very hardy in the environment. Colostral immunity is of utmost importance in the resistance of calves to *C. perfringens* enterotoxemia, since these calves are generally too young to respond to active vaccination. Antibodies against *C. perfringens* and its toxins are passed from dam to calf through colostrum. Calves should consume an adequate amount (about 4 quarts) of high-quality colostrums within the first 18-24 hours of life to gain maximum protection.

Vaccines against clostridial diseases are typically bacterin-toxoids which is meant to stimulate a response against both the bacteria and the toxin produced by the bacteria. Several pre-calving vaccines, called the scour shots contain *C. perfringens* Type C and D bacterin-toxoids. Active vaccination of young calves with *C. perfringens* vaccines such as 7-ways or 2-ways containing Types C and D, or the Type A vaccine is frequently attempted, but little is known about how these vaccines perform in calves less than 1 month of age. Again, these vaccines do not offer protection against the other toxins not included in the vaccine (Glenn and Miskimins 2005).

1.8.7. Black disease

Black disease is thought to occur when there is damage to the liver – such as occurs with migrating liver fluke – that allows *Clostridium novyi* to multiply and produce toxin. The toxin causes severe liver damage and death.

1.8.8. Botulism

Clostridium botulinum is present in decomposing animal and plant material. Toxins are produced by *Clostridium botulinum* in the decaying material. Animals get botulism by ingesting the toxin. The most common source of toxin for cattle is feed contaminated by carcasses such as those of mice or birds, or chewing on bones, the behaviours initiated by phosphorus deficiency. Botulinum toxin causes a flaccid paralysis that starts at the hindquarters and progresses forwards to the forequarters, neck and head. In some cases the tongue is paralysed and hangs from the mouth. The animal is unable to chew or swallow and will drool saliva. Paralysis of the respiratory muscles results in death.

Accidental cases of botulism occur when feed contaminated with rodent, bird or reptile carcasses is fed out. Such contaminated feed should be avoided. In cattle, botulinum vaccine is injected subcutaneously high on the neck. There are two types of vaccine available to prevent botulism *viz.*, a conventional vaccine that requires a booster 4 to 6 weeks after the first dose and a single-dose type that does not require the initial booster. However, both types require an annual booster, as protection only lasts for about 12 months. The time taken to achieve maximum immunity varies from 4 weeks to 6 months. Localised swelling may occur and may take several months to resolve after injecting the vaccine (Prime Fact 440).

References

1. Parker, R., Mathis, C., Looper, M. and Sawyer, J. (2002). Anthrax and livestock. Cooperative Extension Service, College of Agriculture and Home Economics.
2. http://www.doh.sd.gov.
3. http://www.faculty.ccbcmd.edu.
4. Mantur, B. G. and Amarnath, S. K. (2008). Brucellosis in India – a review. *J. Biosci.*, 33: 539-547.
5. Bovine Brucellosis: *Brucella abortus*. The Center for Food Security & Public Health. Iowa State University. www.cfsph.iastate.edu/IICAB. OIE 2009.
6. Elsbach P. (1980). Degradation of microorganisms by phagocytic cells. *Rev. Infect. Dis.*, 2: 106-128.
7. Pizarro-Cerda, J., Meresse, S. and Parton, R. G. (1998). *Brucella abortus* transits through the autophagic pathway and replicates in the endoplasmic reticulum of non-professional phagocytes. *Infect Immun.*, 66: 5711-5724.

8. Anderson, T. D., Cheville, N. F. and Meador, V. P. (1986). Pathogenesis of placentitis in the goat inoculated with *Brucella abortus*. II. Ultrastructural studies. *Vet Pathol.*, 23: 227–239.

9. http://www.sciencephoto.com.

10. Chakraborty, S. (2012). Public Health Importance of Goat Borne Diseases and Zoonoses. LAP LAMBERT Academic Publishing.

11. Fosgate, G. T., Adesiyun, A. A., Hird, D. W., Johnson, W. O., Hietala, S. K., Schurig, G. G. and Ryan, J. (2002). Comparison of serologic tests for detection of Brucella infections in cattle and water buffalo (Bubalus bubalis). *Am. J. Vet. Res.*, 63(11): 1598-1605.

12. Mantur, B. G., Biradar, M. S., Bidri, R. C., Mulimani, M. S., Veerappa, Kariholu, P., Patil, S. B. and Mangalgi, S. S (2006). Protean clinical manifestations and diagnostic challenges of human brucellosis in adults: 16 years' experience in an endemic area; *J. Med. Microbiol.*, 55: 897–903.

13. Kumar, N., Ganguly, I., Singh, R., Deb, S. M., Kumar, S., Sharma, A. and Mitra, A. (2011). DNA polymorphism in SLC11A1 gene and its association with Brucellosis resitance in Indian Zebu (*Bos indicus*) and crossbred (*Bos indicus* X *Bos taurus*) cattle. *Asian-Aust. J. Anim. Sci.*, 24(7): 898-904.

14. Prodinger, W. M., Brandstatter, A., Naumann, L., Pacciarini, M., Kubica, T., Boschiroli, M. L., Aranaz, A., Nagy, G., Cvetnic, Z., Ocepek, M., Skrypnyk, A., Erler, W., Niemann, S., Pavlik, I. and Moser, I. (2005). Characterization of *Mycobacterium caprae* isolates from Europe by mycobacterial interspersed repetitive unit genotyping. *J. Clin. Microbiol.*, 43: 4984–4992.

15. Kirk, J. H. (2002). Tuberculosis in cattle. Extension Veterinarian School of Veterinary Medicine, University of California Davis Tulare, CA.

16. http://www.scientissolutions.com.

17. http://www.pathologyoutlines.com

18. Cousins, D. V. and Florisson, N. (2005). A review of tests available for use in the diagnosis of tuberculosis in non-bovine species. *Rev. sci. tech. Off. int. Epiz.*, 24 (3): 1039-1059.

19. Srivastava, K., Chauhan, D. S., Gupta, P., Singh, H. B., Sharma, V. D., Yadav, V. S., Sreekumaran, Thakral, S. S., Dharamdheeran, J. S., Nigam, P., Prasad, H. K. and Katoch, V. M. (2008). Isolation of Mycobacterium bovis and Mycobacterium tuberculosis from cattle of some farms in North India – Possible relevance in human health. *Ind. J. Med. Res.*, 128: 26-31.

20. Cousins, D. V., Francis, B. R. and Gow, B. L. (1989). Advantages of a new agar medium in the primary isolation of *Mycobacterium* bovis. *Vet. Microbiol.*, 20: 89–95.

21. Gormley, E., Doyle, M. B., Fitzsimons, T., Mc Gill, K. and Collins, J. D. (2006). Diagnosis of *Mycobacterium bovis* infection in cattle by use of the gamma-interferon (Bovigam) assay. *Vet. Microbiol.*, 112 (2–4): 171–179.

22. Griffin, J. F. T., Hesketh, J. B., Mackintosh, C. G., Shi, Y. E. and Buchan, G. S. (1993). BCG vaccination in deer: distinctions between delayed type hypersensitivity and laboratory parameters of immunity. *Immunol. Cell Biol.*, 71: 559–570.

23. Dandliker, W. B., Kelly, R. J., Dandliker, J., Farquahar, J. and Levin J. (1973). Fluorescence polarisation immunoassay: theory and experimental method. *Immunochemistry*, 10 (4): 219-227.

24. Lyashchenko, K. P., Singh, M., Colangeli, R. and Gennaro, M. L. (2000). A multi-antigen print immunoassay for the development of serological diagnosis of infectious diseases. *J. immunol. Met.*, 242 (1-2): 91-100.

25. Greenwald, R., Esfandiari, J., Lesellier, S., Houghton, R., Pollock, J., Aagaard, C., Andersen, P., Hewinson, R. G., Chambers, M. and Lyashchenko, K. (2003). Improved serodetection of *Mycobacterium bovis* infection in badgers (*Meles meles*) using multiantigen test formats. *Diagn. Microbiol. infect. Dis.*, 46 (3): 197-203.

26. Parsons, L. M., Brosch, R., Cole, S. T., Somoskovi, A., Loder, A., Bretzel, G., Van Soolingen, D., Hale, Y. M. and Salfinger, M. (2002). Rapid and simple approach for identification of *Mycobacterium tuberculosis* complex isolates by PCR-based genomic deletion analysis. *J. Clin. Microbiol.*, 40 (7): 2339–2345.

27. Noredhoek, G. T., Van Embden, J. D. A. and Kolk, A. H. J. (1996). Reliability of nucleic acid amplification for detection of *Mycobacterium tuberculosis*: an international collaborative quality control study among 30 laboratories. *J. Clin. Microbiol.*, 34: 2522–2525.

28. Durr, P. A., Hewinson, R. G. and Clifton-Hadley, R. S. (2000). Molecular epidemiology of bovine tuberculosis. I. *Mycobacterium bovis* genotyping. *Rev. sci. tech. Off. int. Epiz.*, 19: 675-688.

29. Kamerbeek, J., Schouls, L., Kolk, A., Van Agterveld, M., Van Soolingen, D., Kuijper, S., Bunschoten, A., Molhuizen, H., Shaw, R., Goyal, M. and Van Embden, J. (1997). Simultaneous detection and strain differentiation of *Mycobacterium tuberculosis* for diagnosis and epidemiology. *J. Clin. Microbiol.*, 35: 907–914.

30. World Health Organization (WHO) / Food and Agriculture Organization of the United Nations (FAO) / Office International des Epizooties (OIE) (1994). Report on Consultation on Animal Tuberculosis Vaccines. WHO, Veterinary Public Health Unit, Geneva. WHO/CDS/VPH/94.138.

31. Vordermeier, H. M., Whelan, A., Cockle, P. J., Farrant, L., Palmer, N. and Hewinson, R. G. (2001). Use of synthetic peptides derived from the antigens ESAT-6 and CFP-10 for differential diagnosis of bovine tuberculosis in cattle. *Clin. Diagn. Lab. Immunol.*, 8 (3): 571-578.

32. Sidders, B., Pirson, C., Hogarth, P. J., Hewinson, R. G., Stoker, N. G., Vordermeier, H. M. and Ewer, K. (2008). Screening of highly expressed mycobacterial genes identifies Rv3615c as a useful differential diagnostic antigen for the *Mycobacterium tuberculosis* complex. *Infect. Immun.*, 76(9): 3932–3939.

33. Deb, R., Saxena, V. K. and Goswami, P. P. (2011). Diagnostic tools against *Mycobacterium avium subspecies paratuberculosis* infection in animals: A review. *Agri Rev.*, 32(1): 46-54.

34. USDA–APHIS. (2006). Uniform Program Standards for the Voluntary Bovine Johne's Disease Control Program (APHIS 91-45-016). Available at: www.aphis.usda.gov/vs/nahps/johnes/.

35. Dargatz, D. A., Byrum, B. A., Barber, L. K., Sweeney, R. W., Whitlock, R. H., Shulaw, W. P., Jacobson, R. H. and Stabel, J. R. (2001). Evaluation of a commercial ELISA for diagnosis of paratuberculosis in cattle. *JAVMA.*, 218(7): 1163-1166.

36. Wells, S. J, Collins, M. T, Faaberg, K. S. (2006). Evaluation of a rapid faecal PCR test for detection of *Mycobacterium avium* subsp. *Paratuberculosis* in dairy cattle. *Clin Vaccine Immunol.*, 13:1125–1130.

37. http://www.sciencedirect.com.

38. Köhler, H., Gyra, H., Zimmer, K., Drager, K. G., Burkert, B., Lemser, B., Hausleithner, D., Cussler, K. and Klawonn, W. (2001). Hess Immune reactions in cattle after immunization with a *Mycobacterium paratuberculosis* vaccine and implications for the diagnosis of *M. paratuberculosis* and *M. bovis* infections. *J. Vet. Med. B*, 48: 185–195.

39. Gilot, P., Dekesel, M., Coene, M. and Cocito, C. (1992). Induction of cellular immune-reactions by A36, an antigen complex of *Mycobacterium paratuberculosis*: comparison of A36 and Johnin components *Scand. J. Immunol.*, 36: 811–821.

40. Burrells, N. F., Inglis, R. C. and Davies, J. M. S. (1995). Detection of specific T cell reactivity in sheep infected with *Mycobacterium avium* subspecies *silvaticum* and *paratuberculosis* using two defined mycobacterial antigens *Vet. Immunol. Immunopathol.*, 45: 311–320.

41. Olsen, L. J., Reitan, G. and Holstad, H. G. W. (2000). Alkyl hydroperoxide reductases C and D are major antigens constitutively expressed by *Mycobacterium avium* subsp. *Paratuberculosis Infect. Immun.*, 68: 801–808.

42. Olsen, P., Boysen, S., Kulberg, J. C., Hope, G. and Jungersen, A. K. (2005). Storset Bovine NK cells can produce gamma interferon in response to the secreted mycobacterial proteins ESAT-6 and MPP14 but not in response to MPB70. *Infect. Immun.*, 73: 5628–5635.

43. Deb, R. and Goswami, P. P. (2010). Expression of a Gene Encoding 34.9 kDa PPE antigen of *Mycobacterium avium* subsp. *paratuberculosis* in *E. coli*. *Mol. Biol. Int.*, vol. 2010, Article ID 628153., 7 pages, 2011. doi: 10.4061/2010/628153.

44. Deb, R. and Goswami, P. P. (2011). Coexpression of PPE 34.9 Antigen of *Mycobacterium avium* subsp. *paratuberculosis* with Murine Interferon Gamma in HeLa Cell Line and Study of Their Immunogenicity in Murine Model. *Biotechnology Research International*, vol. 2011, Article ID 632705, 10 pages, 2011. doi:10.4061/2011/632705.

45. Lombard, J. E., Garry, F. B., Mc Cluskey, B. J. (2005). Risk of removal and effects on milk production associated with paratuberculosis status in dairy cows. *J. Am. Vet. Med. Assoc.*, 227: 1975–1981.

46. Collins, M. T. (1994). Clinical approach to control of bovine paratuberculosis. *J. Am. Vet. Med. Assoc.*, 204: 208–210.

47. Kalis, C. H. J., Hesselink, J. W. and Barkema, H. W. (2000). Culture of strategically pooled bovine fecal samples as a method to screen herds for paratuberculosis. *J. Vet. Diagn. Invest.*, 12: 547–551.

48. Dutta, J., Rathore, B. S., Mullik, S. G., Singh, R. and Sharma, G. C. (1990). Epidemiological studies and occurrence of haemorrhagic septicaemia in India. *Ind. Vet. J.*, 67: 893–899.

49. Kumar, A. A., Harbola, P. C., Rimler, R. B. and Kumar, P. N. (1996). Studies on *Pasteurella multocida* isolates of animal and avian origin from India. *Ind. J. Comp. Microbiol. Immunol. Infect. Dis.*, 17: 120–124.

50. De Alwis, M. C. L. (1990a). Haemorrhagic Septicaemia. ACIAR Monograph No. 57, p. 33.

51. http://ehs.uc.edu.

52. http://www.library.tcmedc.org.

53. Carter, G. R. and Chengappa, M. M. (1980). Hyaluronidase production by type B *Pasteurella multocida* from cases of haemorrhagic septicaemia. *J. Clin. Microbiol.*, 11: 94–96.

54. Boyce, J. D., Chung, J. Y. and Adler, B. (2000). Genetic organisation of the capsule biosynthetic locus of *Pasteurella multocida* M1404 (B:2). *Vet. Microbiol.*, 72: 121-134.

55. Townsend, K. M., Frost, A. J., Lee, C. W., Papadimitriou, J. M. and Dawkins, H. J. S. (1998). Development of PCR assays for species- and type-specific identification of *Pasteurella multocida* isolates. *J. Clin. Microbiol.*, 36: 1096–1100.

56. Verma R. and Jaiswal T. N. (1998): Haemorrhagic septicaemia vaccines. *Vaccine.*, 16: 1184–1192.

57. De Alwis, M. C. L., Wijewardana, T. G., Gomis, A. I. U. and Vipulasiri, A. A. (1990b). Persistence of the carrier state in haemorrhagic septicaemia (Pasteurella multocida serotype 6:B infection) in buffaloes. *Tropic. Anim. Health Prod.*, 22: 185–194.

58. Bolin, C.A. (2003). Diagnosis and control of bovine leptospirosis. Proceedings of the 6th Western Dairy Management Conference. Reno, NV-155.

59. www.aces.edu. Leptospirosis in cattle. Alabama Cooperative Extension System. ANR-0858.

60. Dey, S., Mohan, M., Ramadass, P. and Nachimuthu, K. (2008). Diagnosis of leptospirosis by recombinant antigen based single serum dilution ELISA. *Ind. J. Med. Res.*, 128: 172-177.

61. Faine S. (1982). Guidelines for the control of leptospirosis. WHO Offset Publication No. 67, Geneva.

62. http://www.sciencedirect.com.

63. Dutta, T. K. and Christopher, M. (2005). Leptospirosis – An overview. *JAPI.*, 53: 545-551.

64. Wesley, G. N. (1999). Listeriosis in animals. *In: Listeria*, Listeriosis, and Food Safety, Ryser E. and Marth E., eds. Marcel Dekker, New York, NY, USA, 39–73.

65. Walker, R. L. (1999). Listeria. *In:* Veterinary Microbiology, Hirsh, D. C. and Zee, Y. C., eds. Blackwell Science, Malden, Massachusetts, USA, 225–228.

66. Low, J. C. and Donachie, W. (1997). A review of *Listeria monocytogenes* and listeriosis. *Vet. J.*, 153: 9–29.

67. http://www.811699.net.

68. Quinn, P. J., Carter, M. E., Markey, B. and Carter, G. R. (1999). *Clin. Vet. Microbiol.*, Mosby International, Edinburgh, Scotland, UK.

69. Campero, C. M., Odeon, A. C., Cipolla, A. L., Moore, D. P., Poso, M. A. and Odriozola, E. (2002). Demonstration of *Listeria monocytogenes* by immunohistochemistry in formalin-fixed brain tissues from natural cases of ovine and bovine encephalitis. *J. Vet. Med.*, 49: 379–383.

70. AOAC Official Method 994.03. (2000). *Listeria monocytogenes* in Dairy Products, Seafoods, and Meats. Colorimetric Monoclonal Enzyme-Linked Immunosorbent Assay Method (*Listeria*-Tek). Official Methods of Analysis of AOAC International. *In:* Official Methods of Analysis of AOAC International, Volume I, Agricultural Chemicals; Contaminants; Drugs, Horwitz W., ed. AOAC International, Gaithersburg, MD, USA, 150–152.

71. Gouws, P. A. and Liedemann, I. (2005). Evaluation of diagnostic PCR for the detection of *Listeria monocytogenes* in food products. *Food Technol. Biotechnol.*, 43: 201–205.

72. Graves, L. M., Swaminathan, B. and Hunter, S. (1999). Subtyping *Listeria monocytogenes*. *In: Listeria*, Listeriosis, and Food Safety, Ryser E. & Marth E., eds. Marcel Dekker, New York, NY, USA, 279–297.

73. Salcedo, C., Arreaza, L., Alcala, B., De La Fuente, L. and Vazquez, J. A. (2003). Development of a multilocus sequence typing method for analysis of *Listeria monocytogenes* clones. *J. Clin. Microbiol.*, 41: 757–762.

74. Rudi, K., Katla, T. and Naterstad, K. (2003). Multi locus fingerprinting of *Listeria monocytogenes* by sequencespecific labeling of DNA probes combined with array hybridization. *FEMS Microbiol. Lett.*, 220: 9–14.

75. OIE Terrestrial Manual. (2008). *Listeria monocytogenes*. Chapter 2.9.7. pp. 1238-1254.

76. Robson, S. (2007). Clostridial diseases in cattle. NSW department of primary industries. Prime fact 440. www.dpi.nsw.gov.au.

77. Smith, B. (1996). Large Animal Internal Medicine. pp. 1507-1509. Saint Louis. Mosby-Year Book, Inc.

78. http://www.sdstate.edu.

79. http://www.vet.uga.edu.

80. Williams, B. M. (1977). Clostridial myositis in cattle: bacteriology and gross pathology. *Vet Rec.*, 100: 90-91.

81. Princewell, T. J. T. (1965). Effect of calcium chloride on germination and pathogenicity of *Clostridium chauvoei*. *J. Comp. Pathol.*, 75: 343-351.

82. Naz, S., Ahmad, S. and Bhatti, J. I. (2005). Isolation and identification of Clostridium chauvoei from cattle and buffaloes. *Pak. Vet. J.*, 25(2): 101-102.

83. Daly, R. (2007). *Clostridium perfringens* infections in baby calves. Extension Extra. South Dekota Cooperative Extension Service. ExEx11022.

84. Glenn, S. J. and Miskimins, D. (2005). Clostridial Abomasitis in Calves: Case Report and Review of the Literature. *Anaerobe.*, 11: 290-294.

85. Prime Fact 440. Clostridial diseases in cattle. NSW Department of Primary Industries. www.dpi.nsw.gov.au/primefacts.

□□□

Chapter 2

Major Fungal Diseases of Cattle

Fungi are ubiquitous in nature. There are millions of fungi in nature but only a few of them are established pathogens. However, more and more saprophytic fungi are becoming pathogenic due to disturbances and manipulation in the atmospheric conditions and they are being classified as opportunistic mycoses. In fact, the global picture is quite alarming. During the last three decades the fungal diseases of cattle have been reported four to ten-fold more frequently than before. Fungal diseases are known to occur in all the countries of the world but they occur more commonly in tropical countries like India as fungi in general grow and thrive better in warm and humid conditions. But reports on fungal diseases in India are relatively less than in many developed countries which might be due to lack of awareness and non-availability of proper facilities for diagnosis (Sikdar *et al.*, 2003).

Dermatophytosis, popularly known as ringworm is an example of direct zoonosis. Which affects all species of domestic animals irrespective of age and sex. *Trichophyton verrucosum* is the most common dermatophyte affecting bovines in India (Tewari 1992). Rhinosporidiosis, a chronic, sub-cutaneous fungal infection of man and animals, primarily affecting nasal mucous membrane, characterized by polyploid growth is endemic in certain states of India like Tamil Nadu, Andhra Pradesh, West Bengal and Orissa. In cattle it was first reported by Ayyar (1927). The disease also occurs in equids and water buffaloes. Bullocks suffer more than cows but there is no any influence of sex on the infection (Rao 1938). In South India, the disease runs parallel in man and animals. Although the same species affects both human and animals, there is no evidence of cross infection from man to animal and vice-versa. Candidiasis is another common endogenous infection of man and animals in India. *Candida* spp. have been reported to be responsible for mastitis in cows (Prasad and Prasad 1986) and have also been recovered from aborted foetuses (Monga *et al.*, 1983).

2.1. Dermatophytosis

2.1.1.Introduction

Dermatophytosis, also known as ringworm is an infection of the superficial, keratinized structures of the skin and hair of animals and humans. The disease is caused by a group of keratinophilic, filamentous fungi, called dermatophytes, belonging to the genera *Trichophyton*, *Microsporum*, and *Epidermophyton*.

In cattle, dermatophytosis is most often caused by *T. verrucosum*. Ringworm denotes the clinical entity characterized by annular skin lesions. Although it is a superficial skin infection, ringworm in cattle may have a significant impact on management and economics in affected herds (Deacon 1988).

2.1.2. Etiological agents

In addition to *T. verrucosum*, other species infecting cattle occasionally include *T. mentagrophytes, T. equinum, M. gypseum, M. nanum, M. canis, Keratinomyces ajelloi* and *Chrysosporium* (Nooruddin and Singh 1987). The dermatophytes are molds, characterized morphologically by hyphae forming a mycelium when grown on suitable media. In infected skin, these dermatophytes exist in a parasitic form, characterized by hyphae that may fragment into arthrospores.

2.1.3. Transmission and pathogenesis

Infection occurs by contact with arthrospores or conidia. Infection usually begins in a growing hair or the stratum corneum of the skin. Dermatophytes do not generally invade resting hairs, since the essential nutrients they need for growth are absent or limited. Hyphae spread in the hairs and keratinized skin, eventually developing infectious arthrospores. Transmission between hosts usually occurs by direct contact with a symptomatic or asymptomatic host, or direct or airborne contact with its hairs or skin scales. Infective spores in hair and dermal scales can remain viable for several months to years in the environment. Fomites like brushes and clippers can be important in transmission. Geophilic dermatophytes, such as *M. nanum* and *M. gypseum* are usually acquired directly from the soil rather than from another host.

The dermatophyte antigens are trapped in the epidermis by Langerhans' cells, which are prominent antigen-presenting cells of the skin immune system (Teunissen 1992) and upon exposure to antigens migrate as veiled cells to lymph nodes draining the skin, where the antigens are presented to T-lymphocytes in a major histocompatibility complex (MHC) class II-restricted fashion (Braathen *et al.*, 1983). Granulocyte macrophage-colony stimulating factor (GM-CSF) has been shown to have a stimulatory effect on Langerhans' cells, including potentiation of their antigen-presenting capacity (Kaplan *et al.*, 1992). Different cytokines produced by keratinocytes create favorable conditions in the skin for specific immunological activity (Bos and Kapsenberg 1993). As Langerhans' cells have poor phagocytic capacity, macrophages may have a role in the uptake and degradation of the fungi into smaller fragments. In calves experimentally infected with *T. verrucosum*, an increase in the number of lymphocytes and other inflammatory cells in the dermis *viz.*, macrophages, CD4+ and CD8+ lymphocytes, and yä T cells occurs (Pier *et al.*, 1993). A dense infiltration of neutrophils has been observed in infected areas of the skin in calves experimentally challenged with *T. verrucosum* (Lepper 1974). Phagocytosis and oxidative products of the respiratory burst of neutrophils and macrophages participated in the killing of dermatophytes in vivo. The elimination of dermatophytes is also supported by enhanced epidermopoiesis due to contact sensitivity to fungal elements (Tagami *et al.*, 1989). This leads to an increased turnover of the epidermis, with subsequent elimination of the fungal cells from the skin surface.

2.1.4. Clinical signs

The severity of the disease varies from small focal lesions of 1 cm to extensive generalized skin involvement. The disease often appears as nonpruritic periocular lesions in calves. Cows and heifers may have lesions more often on the chest and limbs, and bulls on the dewlap and intermaxillary skin. The initial lesions are discrete, grayish-white, crusty dry areas with a few brittle hairs. Some areas may become suppurative and thickly crusted. Lesions resembling light brown scabs may also be seen. When these scabs fall off, they leave an area of alopecia. The lesions usually resolve spontaneously in 2 to 4 months.

2.1.5. Diagnosis

Microscopic examination of skin scrapings or hairs in potassium hydroxide (KOH) may reveal hyphae or conidia. A potassium hydroxide-calcofluor white (CFW) mixture can be subjected to fluorescent microscopy to visualize dermatophyte structures. Wood's lamp can be used to examine some strains of *M. canis* that exhibit green fluorescence when stimulated by certain wavelengths of UV light. Definitive diagnosis usually relies on culture. Skin scrapings may be cultured in Dermatophyte Test Medium (DTM) that contains a pH indicator (phenol red) that turns the medium red when a dermatophyte starts growing. Identification is done using a slide culture to observe the reproductive structures (conidia) and hyphae. Species can be identified by the colony structure and colour, microconidia, macroconidia and other microscopic structures (OIE

2005). The cellular response in vaccinated animals can be demonstrated by intradermal injection of the trichophytin 14 days after the 2nd immunization (Mohamed 1989).

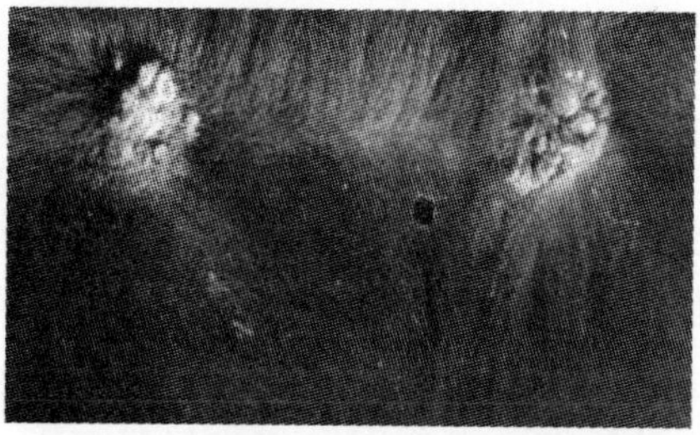

Fig. 12 : Multiple raised pale tan crusted dermatophyte lesion in bovine skin (http://www.vetnext.com).

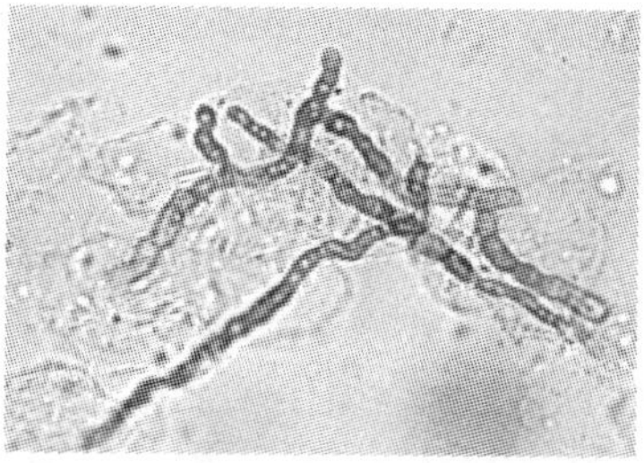

Fig. 13 : KOH mounted infected skin showing typical dermatophyte hyphae http://www.mycology.adelaide.edu.

2.1.6. Prevention and control

Infected animals should be isolated until the infection has resolved to prevent transmission. Animals that have been in contact with the patient should also be checked for asymptomatic infections and antifungals prophylaxis are prescribed for in-contact animals. The premises should be vacuumed and disinfected to help prevent infections in other animals or humans. To prevent the introduction of dermatophytes into herds newly acquired animals should be isolated and cultured.

Live fungal cells were needed to elicit protective immunity. The strain LTF-130 is characterized by abundant production of microconidia and has been used for industrial production of a vaccine (Ringvac bovis LTF-130, Biovet Production, Overhalla, Norway) (Sarkisov 1987) and in Norway. Another vaccine containing an attenuated strain of *T. verrucosum* originates from the former Czechoslovakia (Permavax-Tricho, Bioveta, Ivanovice na Hane, Czech Republic) (Otcenasek *et al.,* 1981).Protective immunity was found to be established 28 d after the 2nd vaccination, and it prevented clinical disease for 1 y after vaccination (Rybnikar *et al.,* 1991). Vaccines for cattle containing formalin-inactivated cells of strains of *T. verrucosum* have also been examined for immunogenicity and protective ability in experimental and field trials (Wawrzkiewicz *et al.*, 1992). Vaccination stimulated a cellular immune response, as assessed by a skin test and a leukocyte migration inhibition test.

2.2. Rhinosporidiosis

Rhinosporidiosis is a chronic disease common o man and animals including cattle and is caused by *Rhinosporidium seeberi*. The disease is characterized by the development of polypoidal granulomatous growth most commonly in the nostrils. The incidence of the disease in cattle population is highest in India. The first case of bilateral nasal form of the disease in India was recorded in bullock and subsequently workers from Kerala, Tamil Nadu and Andhra Pradesh had reported about the occurrence of the disease from time to time (Rao *et al.*, 1975).

The causal organism, once believed to be a protozoan by Seeber is now considered as a fungus belonging to the Phycomycetes. Zschokke (1913) noted close resemblance between human and animal rhinosporidiosis and named the organism as *Rhinosporidium equi*. Subsequently, several names have been proposed and it is now considered that the causative agent is *R. seeberi.*

In Tamil Nadu and Kerala, the disease in man and animals run parallel to each other. In West Bengal, Orissa, Andhra Pradesh, Maharashtra and Madhya Pradesh, human cases are endemic while there are few animal cases. Transmission occurs mostly by direct contact. Ineterestingly, many of the cases of bovine rhinosporidiosis are associated with nasal schistosomiasis (Rao 1938) but the association between the two diseases are yet to be determined (Moses and Balachandran 1987).

The only site of development of infection in animals is nostril. Pedunculated globular growth may develop in the nasal septum along with soft, friable multilobular growth hanging from the turbinate bones along with epistaxis, iching, coughing and post nasal discharge.

Recurrence is common. Sporangia of the organism can be found at post mortem in the nasal cavity.

The organism has not been cultivated in any of the artificial media, natural substrates, chick embryos, tissue culture nor transmitted to experimental animals so far. However, oval shaped fungal sporangia can be demonstrated by impression smears and histopathology. The organisms can be visualized by staining with Periodic Acid Schiff (PAS) as well as Haematoxylin and Eosin (H & E) stain. Potassium chloride preparations can also be used to observe the smears.

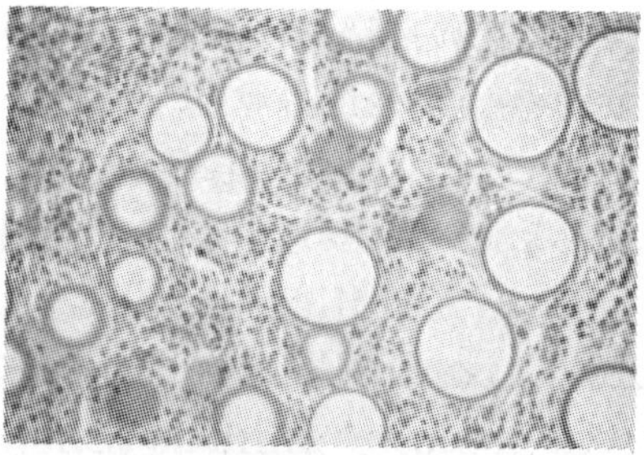

Fig. 14 : Immature trophocytes of *R. seeberi* stained by PAS (http://www.nc. cdc.gov).

In recent years, phylogenetic analysis of the DNA sequences of this organism has made it possible to identify its position in the taxonomic tree along with an organism of medical impotance *Lacazia loboi* (Mendoza *et al.*, 2005). Amphotericin B is the drug of choice for treatment of such craniofacial mycosis. The treatment period varies from 1 to 3 months to prevent recurrence. Because of its high toxicity, the use of this drug for prophylactic purpose is recommended only after confirmed diagnosis (Cohen 1982).

2.3. Candidiasis

Candidiasis is a localized mucocutaneous disease, which is distributed worldwide in a variety of animals, caused by species of the yeast-like fungus, *Candida*, most commonly *C albicans*. *C albicans* is a normal inhabitant of the nasopharynx, GI tract, and external genitalia of many species of animals and is opportunistic in causing disease. Factors associated with candidal infections are disruption of mucosal integrity, indwelling, intravenous, or urinary catheters, administration of antibiotics and immunosuppressive drugs or diseases. Systemic candidiasis occurs in calves apart from mastitis and abortion in adult cattle.

Candida spp. belong to the *Fungi Impevfecti*. They are dimorphic, with a yeast and mycelial phase. In fluid media, the yeast stage predominates, while in tissue, there is a mixed mycelial population. Tissue invasion is often associated with the appearance of mycelial elements (Marrie *et al.*, 1984). In the past, *C. albicans* was assumed to be the only pathogenic yeast of the genus *Candida*. However, it is now known that of the more than 100 species of candida, seven are of medical significance.12 *Candida albicans, C. krusei, C. tropicalis,* and *C. parapsilosis* represent 71 per cent of the *Candida* spp. isolated from domestic animals (Chengappa *et al.*, 1984).

Candida spp. acts as saprophytic guests in the gastrointestinal tract from the first day of life and rapidly becomes parasitic if the environmental balance is compromised for any reason. Signs are variable and non-specific and may be associated more with the primary or predisposing conditions than with the candidiasis itself. Calves with forestomach candidiasis have watery diarrhea, anorexia and dehydration with gradual progression to prostration and death. Bovine abortion due to *Candida* spp. is sporadic in nature. Gross lesions of the skin and mucosae are generally single or multiple, raised, circular, white masses covered with scabs. The organism can penetrate keratinized epithelium and cause marked keratinous thickening of the mucosae of the tongue, esophagus and rumen.

Special stains like Gomori's methenamine silver (GMS), periodic acid-Schiff (PAS), or Brenn and Brown (BB) stain are used to identify yeast organisms as the sole agent consistently associated with lesions. Formalin-fixed tissue can be routinely processed, and ultrathin sections can be examined under transmission electron microscope. The organisms form ger tubes in serum when incubated at 37°C for 2 hours.

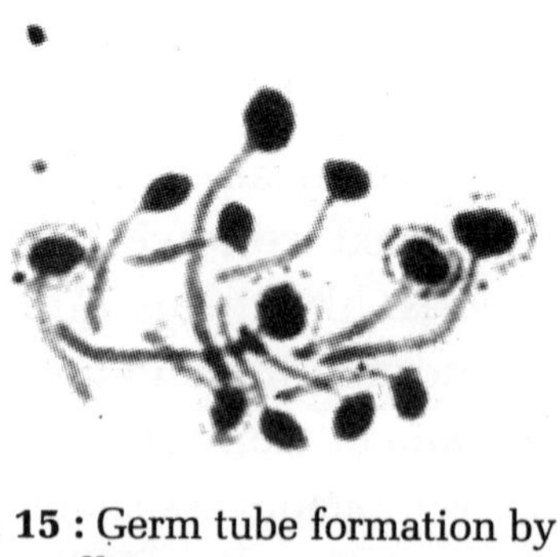

Fig. 15 : Germ tube formation by *C. albicans* in serum demonstrated by Gram's staining http://www.pathmicro.med.sc.edu.

Histopathological examination in case of abortion reveals severe, locally extensive necrotizing placentitis. Overlying trophoblasts show areas of degeneration and necrosis with several small foci of squamous metaplasia and sloughed pyknotic cells. Many of the remaining viable cotyledonary and intercotyledonary trophoblasts reveal numerous, small, 3-4 m diameter yeast organisms within the cytoplasm. Isolation of the organisms can be performed in chocolate agar, trypticase soy agar, Levine EMB, and Columbia CNA (Foley and Schlafer 1987). Nystatin ointment or topical application of amphotericin B or 1% iodine solution may be useful in the treatment of oral or cutaneous candidiasis.

References

1. Sikdar, A., Mullick, S. G. and Ghosh, S. S. (2003). Common fungal diseases of animals in India and their public health importance. www.india veterinarycommunity.com.
2. Ayyar, V. K. (1927). Rhinosporidiosis in cattle. Trans. Far-east Assoc. trop. Med., 3: 658-664.
3. Rao, S. N. (1938). Rhinosporidiosis in bovines in the Madras Presidency, with a discussion on the probable modes of infection. Ind. J. Vet. Sci., 8: 187-198.
4. Prasad, I. B. M. and Prasad, S. (1986). Bovine mastitis caused by an yeast in India. *Vet Rec.*, 79: 809-810.
5. Monga, D. P., Tiwari, S. C. and Prasad, S. (1983). Mycotic abortions in equines. *Mycoses.*, 26(12): 612-614.
6. Deacon, J. W. (1988). Introduction to modern mycology, 2nd ed. Oxford: Blackwell Scientific Publications, pp. 1-239.
7. Nooruddin, M. and Singh, B. (1987). Dermatophytosis in buffaloes, cattle and their attendants. *Mycoses.*, 30(12): 594-600.
8. Teunissen, M. B. M. (1992). Dynamic nature and function of epidermal Langerhans cells in vivo and in vitro: a review, with emphasis on human Langerhans cells. *Histochem. J.*, 24: 697-716.
9. Braathen, L. R. and Kaaman, T. (1983). Human epidermal Langerhans cells induce cellular immune responses to trichophytin in dermatophytoses. *Br. J. Dermatol.*, 109: 295-300.

10. Kaplan, G., Walsh, G., Guido, L. S., Meyn, P., Burkhardt, R. A. and Abalos, R. M. (1992). Novel responses of human skin to intradermal recombinant granulocyte/macrophage-colony-stimulating factor: Langerhans cell recruitment, keratinocyte growth, and enhanced wound healing. *J. Exp. Med.*, 175: 1717-1728.

11. Bos, J. D. and Kapsenburg, M. L. (1993). The skin immune system: progress in cutaneous biology. *Immunol. Today.*, 14: 75-78.

12. Pier, A. C., Ellis, J. A. and Mills, K. W. (1993). Development of immune response to experimental bovine Trichophyton verrucosum infection. *Vet. Dermatol.*, 3: 131-138.

13. Lepper, A. W. D. (1974). Experimental bovine Trichophyton verrucosum infection. The cellular responses in primary lesions of the skin resulting from surface or intradermal inoculation. *Res. Vet. Sci.*, 16: 287-298.

14. Tagami, H., Kudoh, K. and Takematsu, H. (1989). Inflammation and immunity in dermatophytosis. *Dermatologica.*, 179 (1): 1-8.

15. Office des International; Epizootics. (2005). Dermatophytosis. The Center for Food Security and Public Health. pp. 1-6.

16. Mohamed, A. F. (1989). Immunokinetics of experimental dermatophytosis (PhD dissertation). England, Colindale, Mycological Reference Laboratory, pp. 228.

17. http://www.vetnext.com.

18. http://www.mycology.adelaide.edu.

19. Sarkisov, A. K. (1987). Modern methods for control of animal dermatomycosis. *Adv. Agri. Sci.*, Moscow: Nauka, pp. 181-197.

20. Otcenasek, M., Stros, K., Komarek, J., Tomsikova, A., Raskova, H., Hamacek, F. and Zkusenosti, S. (1981). *Vet. Med.*, 26: 193-202.

21. Rybnikar, A., Chumela, J., Vrzal, V. and Krupka, V. (1991). Immunity in cattle vaccinated against ringworm. *Mycoses.*, 34: 433-436.

22. Wawrzkiewicz, K. and Wawrzkiewicz, J. (1992). An inactivated vaccine against ringworm. *Comp. Immun. Microbiol. Infect. Dis.*, 15: 31-40.

23. Rao, P. V. R., Jain, S. N. and Rao, T. V. H. (1975). Animal rhinosporidiosis in India with case reports. *Ann. Soc. Belge. Med. Trop.*, 55(2): 119-124.

24. Zschokke, E. (1913). Ein Rhinosporidium beim Pferde, Schweiz. *Arch. Tierheilkunde.*, 55: 641-650.

25. Rao, M. A. N. (1938). Rhinosporidiosis in bovines in the Madras Presidency, with a discussion on the probable modes of infection. *Ind. J. Vet. Sci.*, 8: 187-198.

26. Moses, J. S. and Balachandran, C. (1987). Rhinosporidiosis in bovines of Kanyakumari district, Tamil Nadu, India. *Mycopathologia.*, 100(1): 23-26.

27. http://www.nc.cdc.gov.

28. Mendoza, L., Viela, R.:, Rosa, P. S. and Fernandez Belone, A. F. (2005). Lacazia loboi and Rhinosporidium seeberi: a genomic perspective. *Rev. Iberoam. Micol.*, 22(4): 213-216.

29. Cohen, J. (1982). Antifungal chemotherapy. *Lancet.*, 2: 532-537.

30. Marrie, T. J., Cooper, J. H. and Costerton, J. W. (1984). Ultrastructure of *Candida parapsilosis* endocarditis. *Infect. Immun.*, 45: 390-398.

31. Chengappa, M. M., Maddux, R. L., Greer, S. C., Pincus, D. H. and Geist, L. L. (1984). Isolation and identification of yeasts and yeast like organisms from clinical veterinary sources. *J. Clin. Microbiol.*, 19: 427-428.

32. http://www.pathmicro.med.sc.edu.

33. Foley, G. L. and Schlafer, D. H. (1987). Candida abortion in cattle. *Vet. Pathol.*, 24: 532-536.

❑❑❑

Chapter 3

Bovine Mastitis

3.1. Introduction

Mastitis (Mast: breast, itis: inflammation) is defined as an inflammatory reaction of udder tissue to bacterial, chemical, thermal or mechanical injury. Mastitis may be either infectious caused by microbial organisms or non-infectious resulting from physical injury to the gland. The inflammatory response consists of an increase in blood proteins and white blood cells in the mammary tissue and the milk. The purpose of the response is to destroy the irritant, repair the damaged-tissue and return the udder to normal function. It is the most costly disease of dairy cattle. About 40% of the cows are infected in an average of two quarters in an herd without an effective mastitis control programme. Reduced milk production accounts for about 70% of the total loss associated with mastitis.

3.2. Impact of mastitis in Indian condition

Bovine mastitis is the most complex disease condition mainly because of multiple causative agents, poor understanding of the early immune response and complexities associated with mammary epithelial cell damage by both the agents and the host factors. Decreased milk production accounts for approximately 70% of the total cost of mastitis. Though, India is the largest milk producer but per capita production is less than half of the world average. Additionally, the poor understanding of the underlying phenomenon in sub clinical state of the infection complicates the therapeutic interventions. It has been observed that about 95% of intramammary infections are caused by *Streptococcus agalactiae, Staphylococcus aureus, Streptococcus dysgalactiae, Streptococcus uberis*, and *Escherichia coli*. The remaining 5% are caused by other organisms. Very comprehensive knowledge of most predominant causative agents and their molecular signature defining the genetic diversity is not available. Further, understanding the disease process emphasizing the contribution of agent and host in the context of modern developments in biological sciences is of paramount importance and this has not been attempted in India, so far. The studies elsewhere in the world have started giving specific insights but the overall understanding is still very poor to arrive at definitive intervention/mitigating strategies. It is in this backdrop, the objectives set out in this research programme will enable us to understand the critical aspects of host-microbe interaction. It will also provide an insight into the intricacies of the progression of the disease so that strategies for rapid diagnosis of sub clinical mastitis can be evolved. In addition, interventions for mitigation of sub clinical and clinical mastitis can be designed and validated for reducing the enormous economic loss incurred due to this disease worldwide. Pathogens invading the mammary gland cause a complex signalling network that activates the early immune defence and leads to inflammation. To examine the importance of mammary epithelial cells in these regulatory pathways, the prime focus is on MEC to infection by specific pathogen. The innate immune response is characterized by the induction of pro-inflammatory cytokines, as well as increases in other accessory proteins that facilitate host recognition and elimination of the pathogens. Thus, the objectives formulated will facilitate better understanding of disease process so that interventions can be designed. But if in case these objectives are not met, the need of the hour will be overlooked and as a consequences, the dairy industry in particular and Indian agriculture as a whole will continue to suffer from huge economic losses. Further, quality of milk has also a great bearing on Public health and such threat to the society will prevail, which will hinder the progress towards making the Indian agriculture globally competitive and ensuring food and nutritional security.

In India, mastitis is a disease with a great economic impact and the estimated loss due to this disease is around Rs. 16,702 millions per annum. Sub clinical mastitis has been found more important in India (varying from 10-50% in cows and 5-20% in buffaloes) than clinical mastitis (1-10%). The incidence was highest in purebred Holsteins and Jerseys and lowest in local cattle and buffaloes. The monsoon season is more suitable for the occurrence of sub clinical mastitis than summer or winter. Prevalence increases with higher lactation number and animals in 4th-5th month of lactation are more susceptible (59.49%) with the characteristic feature of hind quarters being more affected (56.52%) than fore quarters (43.47%). The factors like herd size, agro climatic conditions of the region, variations in socio-cultural practices, milk marketing, literacy level of the animal owner, system of feeding, and management are important in affecting the incidence of sub clinical mastitis. Comparison of efficacy of different diagnostic techniques for sub clinical mastitis, such as Modified California Mastitis Test (MCMT), bromo thymol blue (BTB), modified whiteside test, trypsin inhibition test, milk pH and electric conductivity indicate that MCMT is most sensitive and specific test.

The antimicrobial susceptibility tests have revealed on various occasions that most of the bacterial strains, whether gram positive, gram negative or mixed, isolated from subclinical mastitis milk samples, are highly sensitive to enrofloxacin, least sensitive to oxytetracycline and ampicillin and resistant to streptomycin. The therapy with enrofloxacin and nimesulide are more efficacious in treating sub clinical mastitis in milch cows. Identification of a mastitis pathogen is required for infection study. More than 99% of the mastitis pathogens are bacteria. Sub clinical mastitis is more important in India (varying from 10–50% in cows) than clinical mastitis (1–10%) (Joshi and Gokhale 2006). A number of reports on isolation and characterization of pathogens with special reference to plethora of bacterial species including even *Rhodococcus equi* (Wani *et al.*, 2003), Mycoplasma (Sanjeev Kumar *et al.*, 2005) and fungi (Reports of Monga 1969) are available but few reports of involvement of viruses in mastitis are available so far. Staphylococcus aureus, Streptococcal species and *E. coli* constituted major reported pathogens causing mastitis. Several studies have been conducted in the country from time to time to assess the chemotherapeutic efficacy of antimicrobials, relatedness among various isolates of pathogens like *Staph aureus* and *E. coli* by analysing the dendogram based antibiogram profile and to justify the application of advanced molecular tools like ERIC-PCR in the diagnosis of mastitis.

The IL-2 and IFN-gamma have been expressed in normal healthy cows and diseased cows after *Azadirachta indica* treatment, whereas both the cytokines could not be expressed in cows treated with antibiotic and in untreated diseased cows. The results of the present study indicated anti inflammatory, antibacterial and immunomodulatory potential of the herb (De and Mukherjee 2008). Enhancement of antioxidative and cellular defense and reduction of somatic cell count in the mastitic animals treated with enrofloxacin, vitamin E and selenium as compared to the enrofloxacin treatment alone has been demonstrated in experiments in bovine species with subclinical mastitis (Mukherjee 2008).

3.3. Development of the disease

Mastitis begins after the infectious agent like bacteria pass through the teat duct and enter the cisternal area. Invasion of the teat usually occurs during milking. Organisms present in the milk or at the teat end enter the teat canal and cistern when there is admission of undesired air in the milking unit. After milking, the teat canal remains dilated for 1-2 hours while the canal of a damaged teat may remain partially open permanently. This makes it easier for organisms from the environment or those found on injured skin to enter the teat canal. Adherence of bacteria to tissues lining cisterns and ducts may prevent flushing-out during milking thus helping in establishment of infections. Bacteria eventually enter the glandular tissues where they affect alveolar cells. Toxins produced by bacteria cause either death or damage to milk-secreting epithelial cells and these cells produce substances that circulate in the blood stream and increase blood vessel permeability. This allows leukocytes to move from the blood into the alveolus where they function by engulfing the pathogen.

3.4. Etiological agents

Bacteria are by far the most common cause of mastitis. The most common bacteria include *Streptococcus agalactiae* and *Staphylococcus aureus*. S. agalactiae is the most common cause of sub clinical mastitis but rarely cause acute mastitis. The organism lives inside the cow's udder and survives only for a short time outside the mammary gland. It spreads primarily during milking via the milking machine, and contaminated hands and clothings. *S. aureus* lives inside and outside the udder on the teat skin. The microorganism can cause both clinical and sub-clinical mastitis and spreads the same way as *Strep. agalactiae*. Environmental mastitis is mainly caused by organisms like *Escherichia coli*, *Strep. uberis*, Mycoplasma, *Klebsiella* sp. and *Pseudomonas aeruginosa* that do not normally live in the skin or udder but enter the teat canal when the cow comes in contact with the contaminated environment (Harmon 1994). Yeast like *Candida* sp. can also cause mastitis wherein overuse of antibiotics and poor sanitation contribute to mastitis. Apart from the above organisms, *Arcanobacterium pyogenes* and *Corynebacterium bovis* are associated with Summer mastitis.

3.5. Types of mastitis

Mastitis can be broadly classified as Contagious and environmental mastitis. Contagious mastitis is caused by bacteria that live on the skin of the teat and inside the udder and can be transmitted from one cow to another during milking. The causal agents of environmental mastitis (like *E.coli* as mentioned under the heading Etiological agents) are normally found in feces bedding materials, and feed. Cases of environmental mastitis rarely exceed 10% of the total mastitis cases in the herd.

Contagious mastitis can be divided into three groups *viz.*, clinical, sub-clinical and chronic. Clinical mastitis is characterized by the presence of gross inflammation signs. Three types of clinical mastitis exist *viz.*, per-acute, acute and sub-acute. Per-acute form is characterized by gross inflammation, disrupted functions like reduction in milk yield and changes in milk composition and systemic signs like fever, depression, shivering, loss of appetite and loss of weight. Acute mastitis is similar to the per-acute form but with lesser systemic signs. In case of sub-acute mastitis, the inflammatory signs are minimal and no visible systemic signs are observed. Sub-clinical mastitis is characterized by change in milk composition with no signs of gross inflammation or milk abnormalities. Chronic mastitis for the most part exist as sub-clinical but may exhibit periodical flare-ups in the form of sub-acute or acute form and last for a short period of time. The chronic form may also continue from one lactation to another.

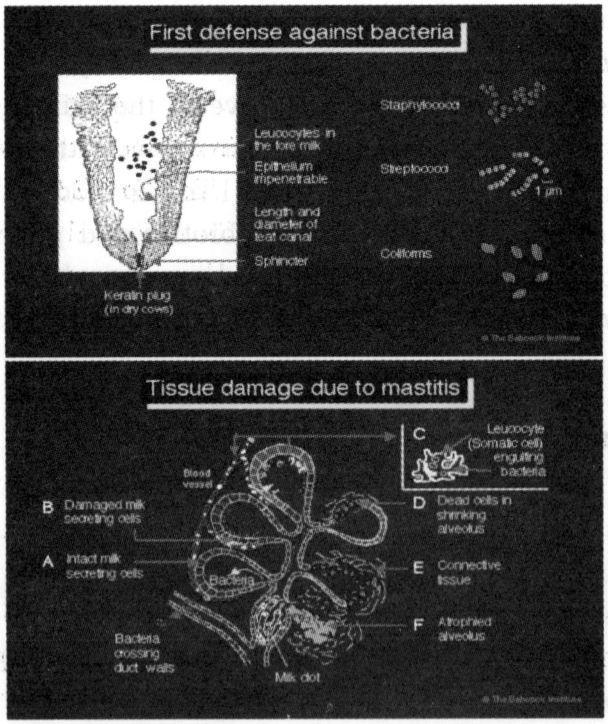

Fig. 16 : Schematic representation of the pathogenesis of mastitis (Courtesy: Dairy Cattle Production 342-450 A)

3.6. Symptoms

Inflammation is characterized by gross abnormalities in the udder *viz.*, swelling, heat, redness, pain. Persisting inflammation leads to tissue damage and replacement of secretory tissues with of the udder with non-productive connective tissues. Abnormalities in milk may include flakes, clots or a watery appearance. The flakes in the milk are congealed leukocytes, secretory cells and protein. Ultimately, there is decreased milk yield.

Table 5 : Changes in milk composition associated with mastitis

Components	Normal milk	Mastitic milk	% of normal
Solid-not-fat	8.98	8.80	99
Fat	35.0	3.20	91
Lactose	4.90	4.40	90
Total protein	3.61	3.56	99
Total casein	2.80	2.30	82
Whey protein	0.80	1.30	162
Serum albumin	0.02	0.07	350
Lactoferrin	0.02	0.10	500
Immunoglobulins	0.10	0.60	600
Sodium	0.06	0.105	184
Chloride	0.09	0.147	161
Potassium	0.17	0.157	91
Calcium	0.12	0.04	33

3.7. Important Diagnostic approaches

3.7.1. Handling of milk sample

The quality of samples for mastitis diagnosis is in many respects more critical than that for many other diseases. Aseptic technique in sample collection for bacterial culturing is an absolute necessity as these same organisms have the potential to cause the disease. Contaminated samples may lead to misdiagnosis. Labelling of samples prior to sampling and including date, farm, cow number and quarter are essential. Using a hand or dry paper towel, loose dirt, bedding and hair from the underside of udder and teats should be brushed.

Discarding a few streams of milk from the quarter and observing milk and udder for signs of clinical mastitis along with predipping all quarters in an effective germicidal predip product and allowing 30 seconds of contact time is of utmost importance. To collect individual quarter samples, sampling should be started from the closest teat towards the teats on the far side of the udder i,e. the reverse order from cleaning. To collect the sample, the cap should be removed from the tube or vial but touching the inner surface of the cap should be avoided. The open end of the cap should always be kept in a downward position. Maintaining the tube or vial at approximately a 45-degree angle while taking the sample is important. Samples should be properly packaged and kept cold at a temperature of less than 40°F or kept frozen during shipping (Waldner 1999).

3.7.2. Cow side testing

3.7.2.1. California Mastitis Test (CMT)

The California Mastitis Test is a simple, inexpensive, rapid screening test for mastitis. The test is based upon the amount of cellular nuclear protein present in the milk sample. Since inflammatory cells associated with mastitis are the predominant cell type present in milk the CMT reflects the SCC level quite accurately and is a reliable indicator of the severity of infection. It is important to understand that a certain percent (around 10-20%) of cows sampled for bacterial culture based on CMT score will have no growth. This is due to a number of factors including short lived infections that have been cleared by the cow or infections that are characterized by intermittent shedding of bacteria like *Strep. agalactiae, Staph aureus* and mycoplasma. The test is appropriate for cow-side evaluation of udder health. The CMT can also be used to evaluate composite milk samples as well as bulk tank milk. In a crisis situation where a herd is at risk of losing it market or quality premiums the test can be used to screen animals or quarters to withhold from the bulk tank. Test criteria for commingled milk are less severe than that for quarter samples because of the dilution effect of milk from normal quarters or cows. It is noteworthy that the value of CMT evaluation of bulk milk decreases as herd size increases.

Table 6 : Relationship between CMT scores and somatic cell count (Jasper 1967)

CMT score	Somatic cell range
N	0-200,000
T	200,000-400,000
1	400,000-1,200,000
2	1,200,000-5,000,000
3	Over 5,000,000

3.7.2.2. R-Mastitest

R-Mastitest is used as indirect test for cow's mastitis diagnosis and it is based on the principle of Californian Mastitis Test (Sargeant *et al.,* 2001). The reagent used in R-Mastitest consists of sodium laurilsulphate, nonylphenol, polyethylene glycol 4000 and bromcresole purple as pH indicator. Homonigenized milk with an equal amount of reagent results in dissolution and rupture of cell and nuclear membranes. This leads to the release of DNA molecules, which will connect and form a gel. The consistency of gel resulted increases as the number of neutrophiles, macrophages, lymphocytes and epithelial cells (in other words the somatic cells) are higher in a mammary quarter.

3.7.2.3. Electrical conductivity

Mastitic milk has a higher electrical conductivity than normal milk due to tissue damage and the subsequent increase in Sodium and Chloride ions in milk. Conductivity sensors are being incorporated in many new automated milking systems. The change in electrical conductivity is one of the earliest manifestations associated with new infections making the routine early detection and recording of possible mastitis cases possible. But the greatest problem associated with this new technology is the sensitivity and specificity of electrical conductivity between herds. However, recent advances in determining herd specific conductivity threshold levels have increased the value of this screening method in many herds. The Mast-O-Test method is a specialised test based on the relationship between milk electrical conductivity and its salt and lactose content (Musser *et al.*, 1998).

3.7.3. Laboratory tests

3.7.3.1. Bulk tank Somatic cell counts (BTSCC)

Bulk tank somatic cell counts (BTSCC) are to be reported to dairy producers on a routine basis usually on bimonthly basis as a measure of milk quality. BTSCC scores can also be used to monitor the level of udder health. In general BTSCC less than 200,000 cells/ml indicate a minimal level of infection, however a series of BTSCC's over 500,000 cells/ml indicate a problem with sub clinical or chronic infection. As the BTSCC is a function of both the quarter infection rate and the severity of infections, attempts to predict the infection status from a single BTSCC proves to be unsuccessful. This is particularly true in case of small herds where an elevated tank count may be the result of exceptionally high counts in a few cows or from a general elevation of counts from many cows.

3.7.3.2. Individual Cow Somatic Cell Counts (SCC)

The most important factor affecting the SCC of milk from a quarter, cow or herd is the infection status of the quarter (Schepers *et al.*, 1997). Individual cow somatic cell counts are the product of the SCC measurement of all milk from all four quarters and the level of production of the individual quarters. Average SCC for uninfected quarters range between 170,000 to 214,000 cells/ml or a geometric mean of 106,000 cells/ml. Somatic cell response of infected cows will depend somewhat on the pathogen present. Minor pathogens such as *C. bovis* and coagulase-negative *Staphylococcus* average 227,000 cells/ml when all age groups are considered. Animals infected with major pathogens like *Streptococcus agalactiae, Staphylococcus aureus* or Environmental *Streptococci* produce average counts greater than

600,000 cells/ml. The number of infected quarters as well as the total milk production become important factors in being able to accurately classify a cow as infected by means of SCC. The dilution effect of normal milk can mask infection.

3.7.3.3. Linear score

Official test scores of somatic cell counts are typically reported as Log linear scores of the raw SCC. Log linear scores provide a more accurate and direct measure of milk losses associated with increasing SCC. The average LS give a less distorted and more accurate picture of a lactation than does the average raw SCC. For these reasons linear score is used most frequently when analyzing and graphing SCC data.

Table 7 : Relationship between SCC linear score (LS) and Somatic cell count (SCC) range (Shook and Seaman 1983)

LS	SCC range
O	0-18,999
1	19,000-35,999
2	36,000-71,999
3	72,000-1,41,999
4	1,42,000-2,83,999
5	2,84,000-5,65,999
6	5,66,000-1,130,999
7	1,131,000-2,262,999
8	2,263,000-4,523,999
9	4,524,000 - >9,999,999

3.7.3.4. Culturing of milk

Culturing milk from the bulk tank, individual quarter or cow, groups or categories of cows helps in adding an additional dimension to evaluating udder health and mastitis control programs especially when the information is combined with SCC or clinical mastitis data. Routine milk cultures is an important component of any mastitis control program. Sampling the bulk tank milk (BTC) is a simple, inexpensive means of determining the presence of mastitis pathogens in a herd. This culturing method is best suited for the identification of contagious mastitis pathogens and for monitoring the presence of pathogens over time. BTC from herds with a low prevalence of infection with a specific organism, especially contagious pathogens like *Staphylococcus aureus, Streptococcus agalactiae* and *Mycoplasma* spp. may not always indicate the presence of those pathogens. Hence, BTC results should always be considered when collected as a series of tests over a given period of time.

3.7.3.5. Individual animal culture

Individual animal cultures provide another method of diagnosing mastitis. Cultures alone provide an indication of the possible pathogen involved. However the possibility of a false positive result due to contamination of the sample with organisms present in the teat canal, teat skin or environmental contamination of the sample can affect test specificity. Individual cow culture results become much more meaningful when combined with SCC results. Using SCC to select cows at high risk to be sampled for milk culture ensures a relatively good predictive value for the culture results. Using two tests simultaneously to evaluate animals increases the sensitivity but causes slight decrease in the specificity. Predictive value (PV) of a test is defined as the proportion of infected animals among those that are test positive. The predictive value of any given test is a function of the test specificity, sensitivity as well as the prevalence of the disease in the herd. The predictive value of a test decreases as the prevalence of the disease decreases within the herd. When applied to SCC and milk cultures the specificity of culture results improves as the SCC threshold increases. In most herd investigations using an LS of 4.0 (SCC = 200,000 cells) provides approximately 70 to 80 % sensitivity and specificity.

3.7.3.6. Capture immunoassays using monoclonal antibodies

A direct capture enzyme-linked immunosorbent assay (ELISA) can be used to measure elevated polymorphonuclear granulocyte

(PMN) antigens using horseradish peroxidase conjugated rabbit polyclonal anti-PMN antisera and a monoclonal antibody specific for PMN cells. Optical densities obtained in the ELISA are useful to predict the cell counts of milk samples (O'Sullivan *et al.*, 1992).

3.7.3.7. DNA approach

DNA amplification of the target pathogen by PCR even though is more expensive than culture method, but the efficiency and accuracy of pathogen identification is high. Million to billion fold amplification of the targeted DNA sequence can be achieved by using pathogen specific probes. For instances, the use of Pathoproof Mastitis PCR assay for amplification of the staphylococcal beta-lactamase gene has gained popularity in recent years. By this assay pathogen identification can be done within 4 hours. The use of diagnostic kits like MasTest helps in health monitoring and breeding for mastitis resistance as such kits can detect pathogen related variability in heritability and aids in selection of marker genes. Automated quantitative real time PCR (qRT-PCR) is fast, accurate and helps in quantitative detection of pathogen upto species level (Report of Bredbacka and co-workers).

3.7.4. Computerized herd record analysis

Use of computerized herd record analysis programs such as Dairy Comp 305 allows management to be more proactive in dealing with udder health and issues involving milk quality. Monitoring can also serve as a motivational tool and marketing device for quality milk technical services. Producers who enter other disease and health data into Dairy Comp can also evaluate the incidence and prevalence of clinical mastitis the possible interaction other health problems such as metabolic disease, DA, retained placenta etc with udder health (NYSCHAP reports).

3.8. Prevention and control

Measures aiming at preventing new cases of mastitis from occurring include breeding, improvement of milking hygiene, implementation of post-milking teat disinfection, regular controls of the milking equipment, implementation of milking order, and improvement of bedding material. Antibiotic treatment protocols, dry cow therapy, and culling regimes are examples of actions that are taken in order to limit the impact of mastitis once it has occurred (Nielsen 2009). When a herd problem is faced, the proper sampling method to employ should be determined in accordance with the history of the herd and the urgency of the situation. Herds with a history characteristic of contagious mastitis such as a steady rise in BTSCC or those highly suspect of having contagious mastitis may benefit from an initial bulk tank culture. Any herd known to have contagious mastitis caused by *Staphylococcus aureus, Streptococcus agalactiae* or *Mycoplasma* spp. with an interest to eliminate the infection from the herd must have a whole herd survey. A whole herd survey provides an estimate of infection prevalence or an inventory of mastitis pathogens in a herd. A single survey provides an excellent estimation of the herd prevalence rate of specific pathogens. When elimination of a contagious pathogen such as *Strep. agalactiae* becomes a herd goal, frequent herd surveys become necessary. Success of such a program is heavily dependant upon accurate identification of infected animals so that infection can be contained by means of segregation of infected animals at milking time as well as effective treatment of the infected animals. A delay in the time interval between surveys will allow the infection to spread, hindering the eradication process and increasing the associated costs. Such principle of conducting quick and accurate survey apply to the contagious pathogens such as *Staphylococcus aureus* and *Mycoplasma* spp. Mycoplasma infections are untreatable. Infected cows can remain infected for life, become intermittent shedders and are a constant source of new infections. Culling infected cows provides the most effective means of infection control. *Staph aureus* infection is also very difficult to cure. This is particularly true for treatment during lactation. Treatment at dry off offers a greater opportunity to eliminate infections but *Staph aureus* infection too frequently carry through to the next lactation. Producers with relatively low levels of infection or low BTSCC can be benefitted from milk cultures of problem animals. Milk cultures based on stage of lactation or history can provide valuable information concerning pathogen prevalence, monitoring the effectiveness of control programs or treatment protocols and is used to identify risk factors for new infection. For instance, the dry period is a known risk factor for new infections by environmental pathogens. Environmental *Streptococci* and coliform infections are 2 to 12 time more likely to occur during the dry period than lactation. To provide a better understanding of the new infection rate during the dry period a producer can use linear score to select cows for sampling and possible treatment. A producer not taking advantage of computerized herd record analysis data can use CMT results to reach similar conclusions. A similar testing method can be used to samples cows at dry off to identify quarters of the infected cows, evaluate the effectiveness of dry cow treatment or use selective dry cow therapy. Culturing clinical quarters can provide valuable information concerning pathogen prevalence and provide a more logical means of selecting appropriate treatment protocols. When used in conjunction with SCC and other production parameters the data can provide valuable insight for identifying risk factors such as stage of lactation, low SCC, parity, or production group and provide a basis for evaluating the effectiveness of vaccination programs or treatment methods.

Considering that most cows in a herd are of second or later parities and that SCC is highest in multiparous cows, the majority of the production loss caused by mastitis is likely to be experienced by multiparous cows. Thus, special emphasis should be put on reducing the incidence of mastitis in multiparous cows. This can be attempted by enhanced mastitis control in primiparous cows because cows that have suffered from mastitis are more likely to develop subsequent cases. Attention should be paid to cows in early and late stages of lactation. During these periods, the incidence of mastitis is highest and yield losses are most severe, but, by taking proper actions, unnecessary milk loss can be avoided. The frequency of mastitis in the dairy cow population can also be decreased by breeding for cows with better ability to resist udder disease. Udder health is unfavourably genetically correlated with milk yield (Carlen *et al.*, 2004), and selecting only for increased production, which traditionally has been the focus of dairy cattle breeding. This can be counteracted by applying a broad breeding goal which includes not only production traits, but functional traits such as mastitis resistance. The genetic progress in a trait is partly determined by the relative weight put on it in the total merit index of bulls. In order to assign proper economic weight to mastitis resistance, accurate estimates of the economic loss caused by mastitis are necessary (Carlen 2008).

3.8.1. Understanding the genetics of mastitis susceptibility

Breeding for resistance to udder pathogens is an important tool. Periparturient mastitis susceptibility is related to the generalized immune suppression taking place from approximately 1 week prepartum to approximately 1 week postpartum. Thus, it is necessary to identify the genes responsible for such condition. Genetic selection against periparturient mastitis susceptibility may be the best long-term approach. The global gene expression changes occurring in bovine blood leukocytes around parturition has been done by cDNA microarray analysis. However, it has not been determined which population of leukocytes are affected or what factors of parturition cause the repression of the leukocyte genes (altogether 18 genes have been identified by microarray experiment). A majority of them showed high DNA sequence homology to genes that are needed for normal cell functions (Burton *et al.*, 2003). The new finding in the gene expression studies include the identification of the gene that produces a protein that is naturally present in cows' milk and blood plasma but in an amount too small to have any therapeutic effect. The recombinant protein, named CD14 binds to and neutralizes endotoxins that are made by bacteria causing mastitis. Studies are now being conducted to support the new hypothesis that cows genetically engineered to produce higher than normal amounts of CD14 can get protection from infection as well. Moreover, numerous experiments have identified different QTL regions in cattle. These QTLs envelop large chromosomal regions on average spreading from 10 to 40 cM which involve hundreds or thousands of genes. The goal of QTL analysis is identification of the causal gene itself. Besides QTLs, a large number of genetic polymorphisms within the causal gene regions or genetic markers associated with mastitis traits have also been identified in cattle by microarray analysis. New knowledge regarding the genetics of mastitis susceptibility ultimately helps in the development of novel management strategies.

References

1. Joshi, S. and Gokhale, S. (2006). Status of mastitis as an emerging diseases in improved and periurban dairy farms in India. *Annals of The New York Acad. Sci.*, doi: 10.1196/annals.1373.007.
2. Wani, S. A., Bhat, M. A., Qureshi, S. and Bachh, A. S. (2003). Isolation of *Rhodococcus equi* from clinical bovine mastitis – A case report. *Ind. J. Anim. Res.*, 37(1): 75-76.
3. Sanjeev Kumar, M., Murag, S. and Hari Babu, Y. (2005). Biochemical and immunological identification of mycoplasma isolates from bovine mastitis. SRDDL, Institute of Animal Health and Veterinary Biologicals, Hebbal, Bangalore.
4. Monga, D. P. (1969). Studies on mastitis due to fungi and *mycoplasma* in domestic animals. Under the guidance of Dr. D. S. Kalra.
5. De, U. K. and Mukherjee, R. (2008). Anti-inflammatory and respiratory burst activity of *Azadirachta indica* during acute bovine mastitis. *Ind. J. Anim. Sci.*, 79(2): 32-34.
6. Mukherjee, R. (2008). Selenium and Vitamin E increases polymorphonuclear cell phagocytosis and anti-oxidant levels during acute mastitis in riverine buffaloes. *Vet. Res. Commun.*, 32(4): 305-313.
7. Harmon, R. J. (1994). Mastitis and genetic evaluation for somatic cell count – Physiology of mastitis and factors affecting somatic cell counts. *J. Dairy. Sci.*, 77(7): 2103-2112.

8. Dairy Cattle Production 342-450A. Mastitis in dairy cows. Faculty of Agricultural and Environmental Sciences. Department of Animal Science. Mac Donald Campus of Mac Gill University.

9. Waldner, D. N. (1999). Bovine mastitis: Milk sample collection and handling. Division of Agriculturl Sciences and Natural Resources. Oklahoma State University. Oklahoma Cooperative Extension Fact Sheets. http://osufacts.okstate.edu.

10. Jasper, D. E. (1967). Proceedings of National Masitis Council (adapted).

11. Sargeant, J. M., Leslie, K. E., Shirley, J. E., Pulkrabek, B. and Lim, G. H. (2001). Sensitivity and specificity of somatic cell count and California Masititis Test for identifying intramammary infection in early lactation. *J. Dairy Sci.*, 84: 2018-2024.

12. Musser, J. M. B., Anderson, K. L. and Caballero, M. (1998). Evaluation of a hand-held electrical conductivity meter for detection of subclinical mastitis in cattle. *Am. J. Vet. Res.*, 59: 1087-1091.

13. Schepers, A. J., Lam, T. J. G. M., Schukken, Y. H., Wilmink, J. B. M. and Hanekamp, W. J. A. (1997). Estimation of variance components for somatic cell counts to determine thresholds for uninfected quarters. *J. Dairy Sci.*, 80(8): 1833-1840.

14. Shook, G. and Seaman, A. (1983). *JDS.*, 39(12).

15. O'Sullivan, C. A., Joyce, P. J., Sloan, T. and Shattock, A. G. (1992). Capture immunoassay for the diagnosis of bovine mastitis using a monoclonal antibody to polymorphonuclear granulocytes. *J. Dairy Res.*, 59(2): 123-133.

16. Bredbacka, P., Salmikivi, L. and Koskinen, M. T. Next-day results in bovine mastitis diagnostics using DNA technology and electronic reporting. Finnzymes Diagnostics.

17. New York State Cattle Health Assurance Programme (NYSCHAP) Veterinary Resource. Diagnosis of mastitis and diagnostic methods for investigating udder health problems.

18. Nielsen, C. (2009). Economic impact of mastitis in dairy cows. Doctoral Thesis. Swedish University of Agricultural Sciences, Uppsala, Sweden.

19. Carlen, E., Strandberg, E. and Roth, A. (2004). Genetic parameters for clinical mastitis, somatic cell scores, and production in the first three lactations of Swedish Holstein cows. *J. Dairy Sci.*, 87(9): 3062-3070.

20. Carlen, E. (2008). Genetic evaluation of clinical mastitis in dairy cattle. Doctoral Thesis. Swedish University of Agricultural Sciences, Uppsala, Sweden.

21. Burton, J. L., Madsen, S. A., Yao, J., Sipkovsky, S. S. and Coussens, P. M. (2003). An immunogenomics approach to understanding periparturient immunosupression and mastitis susceptibility in dairy cows. *Acta. Vet. Scand.*, 98: 71-88.

□□□

Chapter 4

Major Viral Diseases of Cattle

The relationship between viral disease in cattle and the state of underdevelopment can be studied in the light of the process of dependence existing in the world economic order between countries that produce industrial goods and the group of countries which, as producers of raw materials that include animal protein, comprise the underdeveloped periphery of the world economic order (Astudillo and Rosenberg 1983). In this context, viral diseases are factors which contribute to create the status of underdevelopment, but may also be consequences of that very underdevelopment—a state that in many cases explains the introduction and dissemination of such diseases, as well as the difficulties encountered in developing countries like India in controlling them. The impact of viral diseases on foreign trade is also very important, mostly because of animal health restrictions based on endemic diseases like foot and mouth disease and infectious bovine rhinotracheitis. Moreover, the lethal diarrhea of calves caused by rota viruses and of course the zoonotic disease like rabies are quiet noteworthy. Finally, the development of the livestock industry in India is hampered by a low capability for prevention of viral diseases because of weakness of epidemiological surveillance mechanisms and absence or lack of a suitable number of adequate diagnostic laboratories. Once deadly plague of cattle, the Rinderpest, has been eradicated from India during the year 2006 (as declared by the national newspaper The Hindu on 9th July, 2006) and so also globally and its official declaration had been made on 23rd

August, 2011 by the Indian Council of Agricultural Research. Thus, research and development on viruses with respect to the epidemiology, diagnosis, pathogenesis and vaccinology of virus infections need to be strengthened, an international network of databases of virus infections needs to be instituted and a global network for the diagnosis and containment of viral diseases is advocated (Banerjee 1996) for containment and subsequent eradication of the other major infectious diseases of cattle prevalent in India.

4.1. Foot-and-mouth disease (FMD)

4.1.1. Introduction

Foot-and-mouth disease (FMD) is a highly contagious disease affecting *artiodactylae* including cattle (Brooksby 1982). FMD affects extensive areas worldwide and is included in the list of diseases notifiable to the World Organization for Animal Health. It is recognized as a significant epidemic disease threatening the cattle industry since the sixteenth century and till date it is a major global animal health problem. The disease is endemic in India since many centuries. It is present almost in all parts of the country and occurs round the year. Approximately 470 million domestic livestock including cattle are susceptible to FMD apart from the free-living and captive wild ungulates.

Even though FMD involves mortality rates below 5%, but still it is considered as the most important disease of farm animals since it causes huge losses in terms of livestock productivity and trade. Although Foot-and-mouth disease virus (FMDV) rarely causes death in adult animals, the virus can cause severe lesion in the myocardium of young animals, leading to high mortality rates (Woodbury 1995). The main constraints in controlling this disease and the reasons for considering it as the most dreaded viral disease are its high contagiousness, wide geographical distribution, broad host range, ability to establish carrier status, antigenic diversity leading to poor cross-immunity, and relatively short duration of immunity. Poor surveillance and diagnostic facilities as well as inadequate control programs are major problems in control of this disease in the country. FMD is still a leading cause of loss of livestock economy in India. Outbreaks are still being reported from time to time around the year (Tamilselvan *et al.*, 2009). There are records of about 5,000 outbreaks to occur in India annually affecting nearly three lakh animals with an estimated staggering loss of Rs. 4,300 cores to the economy annually.The losses are mainly due to reduction in milk yield, draught power, and breeding capabilities. In India where world' largest livestock populations exist, it is a leading cause of loss of livestock economy (direct and indirect losses) due to its endemic nature (Longjam *et al.*, 2011). Besides causing direct losses to livestock economy it also causes indirect losses in terms of severe trade restrictions, impact which may be higher than direct losses.

4.1.2. Etiological agent and its serotypes

The etiological agent, foot-and-mouth disease virus (FMDV) is classified within the genus *Aphthovirus* in the family *Picornaviridae* (Racaniello 2001). The virus exists in the form of seven serologically and genetically distinguishable types, namely, O, A, C, Asia1, SAT1, SAT2, and SAT3, but a large number of subtypes have evolved within each serotype (Pereira 1977). Out of the possible seven, only four serotypes, *viz.*, O, A, C and Asia 1 were ever recorded in India. Serotype C too has not been recorded in the country since 1995. Of the different serotypes prevalent in India, type O has been found to be predominant over other types (Ahuja *et al.*, 1996). Similarly in the North-Eastern region of India, the frequency of FMD is highest with type O which is always followed by other types including the type Asia-1 (Sarma *et al.*, 1992). It has been recorded that about 85% of the outbreaks of FMD in India are caused by serotype 'O', followed by 'A', which account for about 8 to 10% and the rest due to Asia 1. It has also been established that out of a possible ten genotypes of serotype 'A', only two, *i.e.*, VI and VII are circulating in India for the last 20 years. In Asia 1 too genotypes VIA and VIB are co-circulating in India. Molecular epidemiology of FMD by nucleotide sequencing of the 1D gene and/or the entire P1 region forms the basis of such genotyping (Reports of Bandyopadhyay, I.V.R.I).

4.1.3. Structure and genomic organization of FMDV

The virion contains a single-stranded RNA of positive polarity, approximately 8500 nucleotides long. It is an icosahedral particle with a smooth surface and a diameter of about 30nm. There are 60 copies of each of the structural protein VP1, VP2, VP3, and VP4. While the first three structural proteins (having molecular weight of 24 kDa) have surface components, the fourth (having molecular weight of 8.5 kDa) is internal. The virion also contains one or two units of VP0, the precursor of VP2 and VP4. The structural proteins *viz.,* VP1-3 fold into an eight-stranded wedge-shaped 13-barrel which fits together to form the majority of the capsid structure. The three-dimensional structure of FMDV has revealed a prominent surface feature formed by the loop between the G and H strands of VP1. The VP4 protein is located inside the capsid. The strands of the 13-barrel of VP1-3 are connected by loops which form the outer surface of the virion (Bachrach 1968; Acahrya *et al.,* 1989). Unlike other picornaviruses, FMDV lacks a surface canyon or pit which is the receptor binding site for entero- and cardioviruses. Another feature of the virion is the channel at the fivefold axis which permits the entry of small molecules such as Cscl into the capsid resulting in FMDV having the highest buoyant density of the picornaviruses [42]. The main cell attachment site and the immunodominant region of FMDV are both located on a solvent exposed region at the surface of the virion, namely, in trypsin-sensitive areas of VP1. Earlier serological studies showed that different serotypes of FMDV shared a highly variable region of VP1 as one of the major antigenic sites of the virus (Strohmaier *et al.,* 1982).

The genome of FMDV is about 8.5 Kb in length enclosed within a protein capsid. It has four major parts *viz.,* 5' Untranslated region (5' UTR), Coding region, 3' Untranslated region (3' UTR), and a poly "A" tail. The 5' UTR is linked with Vpg (3B) which serves as primer in replication. 5' UTR contains an S fragment at its 5' end which encompasses 360 bases, folds into long stem loop and plays a role in genome stability and the binding of protein involved in genome replication. Following S fragment there is poly "C" tract comprising over 90% "C" residues. The length of this tract is extremely variable. There are some evidences that length of this tract is associated with virulence and hence persistence. After poly "C" tract, there is a series of RNA pseudo knot structures of unknown function. Downstream to the pseudo knot there is cisacting replicative element (cre). The cre has conserved AAA sequences and is essential for genome replication. Downstream to cre is internal ribosomal entering sites (IRES). The IRES has role in initiation of viral protein synthesis and shutting down of host cell protein synthesis (Mason *et al.*, 2002; Grubman and Baxt 2004). Due to the presence of IRES, FMDV can bind to ribosomes to initiate the protein synthesis.The picornaviruses have no 5' cap (7-methyguanosine), so IRES serves as ribosomal entering site. The 3' UTR follows the ORF (open reading frame) termination codon and contains a short stretch of RNA which folds into specific stem loop structures followed by a poly "A" tract of variable length. This 3' UTR also serves some functions in genome replication. Poly "A" probably plays a role in FMDV translation and replication (Lopez *et al.*, 2002). The FMDV genome encodes a polyprotein from which four different structural and eight different non-structural proteins are formed by the viral proteases. FMDV has two proteinases. The NSP leader proteinses (Lpro) located in the N-terminal region of the polyprotein acts both intra and intermolecularly. This protease initiates cleavage by separating itself from P1, the precursor of the capsid protein and the remainder of the growing polypeptide chain. The 3C protease is responsible for the cleavage of P1 into 1AB (VP0), 1C (VP3), and 1D (VP1). The 1A/1B (VP4/VP2) cleavage occurs at the late stage in virus morphogenesis and is associated with maturation of capsid. The 2C/3A primary cleavage is cis and subsequent cleavage is also mediated by the 3Cpro and producing processing intermediates and mature proteins. In addition to viral protein processing, the 3Cpro cleave the host cell protein histone H3 andmay be involved with the shutting down of host cell transcription (Ryan *et al.*, 1991).

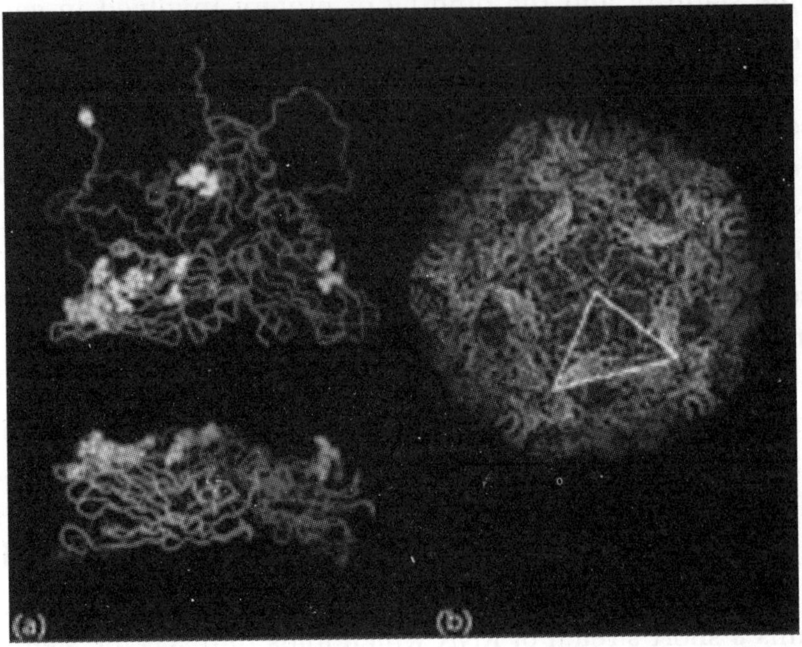

Fig. 17 : Structure of foot-and-mouth disease virus. The capsid is built from four viral structural proteins, VP1–4. **(a)** Shows a mature protomer, the smallest repeating unit, contains one copy of each of VP1–3; Blue, VP1; Green, VP2; Yellow, VP3. Sidechains of amino acids that are targeted by neutralizing antibodies are shown in white on the peptide backbone of the protomer. Upper image is viewed from above; lower image is viewed through the plane of the capsid. **(b)** The capsid. Five protomers (triangle=one protomer) assemble into a saucer-shaped, pentagonal disc, with VP1 in the centre. Twelve of these pentamers make a complete capsid. VP4 is not shown since it is entirely internal within the capsid (http://www.els.net).

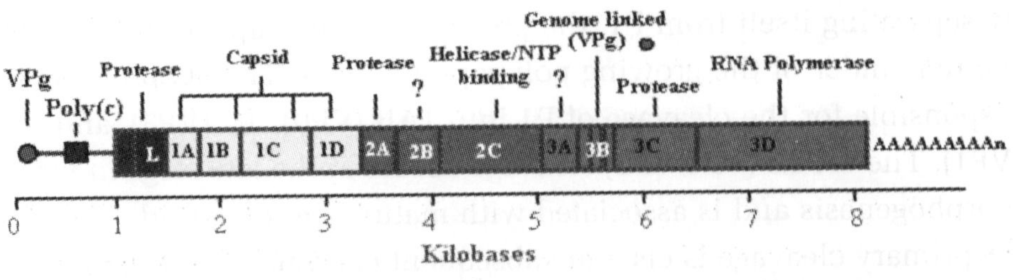

Fig. 18 : Genome map of FMDV (http://www.foot-and-mouth.org).

4.1.4. Epidemiology

FMD is a highly transmissible disease and a limited number of infective particles can initiate host infection (Sellers 1971). Contaminated animal products, nonsusceptible animals, agricultural tools, people, vehicles, and airborne transmission (Donaldson *et al.*, 1987) can contribute to the mechanical dissemination of the virus. The epidemiology of FMD is complex, and it is affected by different viral, host, and environmental factors. Among them, variations in virus virulence (severity of lesions, amount, and duration of virus release), particle stability in different microenvironments, and chances of long-term persistence are important. FMDV multiplication and spread also depend on the host species, nutritional and immunological status, population density, animal movements, and contacts between different domestic and wild host species and animals capable of mechanical dissemination of the virus (Nishiura and Omori 2010). The environment can provide geographical barriers to virus dissemination or, alternatively, can promote virus transmission when appropriate atmospheric conditions prevail. In this multifactorial scenario (Ferguson *et al.*, 2001), the high potential for FMDV variation and adaptation hasmodelled complex evolutionary patterns that are being revealed by molecular epidemiology analyses, mostly based on nucleotide sequencing of capsid protein genes. The agroclimatic and socioeconomic condition, mixed animal husbandry practices, unrestricted movement, and trade among animals and porous international border provide a conductive epidemiology niche for the FMDV to flourish, mutate, and persist over time and to affect the susceptible animal population (Mishra *et al.,* 1998).

4.1.5. Pathology and pathogenesis

FMDV produces an acute and systemic vesicular disease. In natural infection, the main route of virus entry is the respiratory tract. Initially, the virus multiplies in the pharyngeal epithelium, producing primary vesicles, or "aphthae" (Burrows *et al.,* 1981). The vesicles produced by FMDV generally affect cells of the stratum spinosum layer. The clinical outcome of the disease may vary among the infecting virus strain. Fever and viraemia usually start within 24–48 hr after epithelium infection, leading to viral spread into different organs and tissues and the production of secondary vesicles preferentially in the mouth and feet. The acute phase of disease lasts about 1 week and declines gradually coinciding with the emergence of a strong humoral response (Salt 1993). The morbidity and mortality in FMD depends upon the breed and age of the animal where mortality in adult animals is as low as 2 per cent in comparison to 20 per cent in young stock (Radostits *et al.,* 1994). The calves show prominent signs of myocarditis, whereas piglets manifest gastroenteritis (Buxton and Fraser 1977). Asymptomatic, persistent infection can also be established during which infectious virus can be isolated from the oesophagus and throat fluids of the animals from a few weeks up to several years of the initial infection. There is epidemiological evidence to support the hypothesis that carrier animals may be the origin of outbreaks of acute disease when brought into contact with susceptible animals. This mode of transmission has been experimentally reproduced for serotype SAT isolates (Vosloo *et al.,* 1996).

4.1.6. Diagnosis

The accurate diagnosis of infection with FMDV is of prime most importance for both control and eradication campaigns in FMD endemic areas and as a supportive measure to the stamping out policy in FMD-free areas (Remond *et al.,* 2002). Presently FMD diagnosis is being carried out using techniques such as Virus Isolation, Sandwich-ELISA, Liquid-Phase Blocking ELISA (LPBE), Multiplex-PCR (m-PCR), indirect ELISA (DIVA) along with real time-PCR which can be used for detection of antibody against non-structural proteins. Nucleotide sequencing for serotyping, microarray as well as recombinant antigen-based detection, biosensor, phage display, and nucleic-acid-based diagnostic are on the way for rapid and specific detection of FMDV. Various pen side tests, namely, lateral flow, RT-LAMP and immunostrip tests are also developed for detection of the virus in field condition.

4.1.6.1. Virus isolation

The most sensitive culture system for virus isolation is primary bovine thyroid cells but cryo-preservation of bovine thyroid cells directly after trypsinization results in the loss of susceptibility to FMDV. Some stable cell lines, like IBRS-2, MVPK-1 clone 7, LFBK cell line and BHK-21 are also susceptible to FMDV and so are most desirable for diagnostic system but these are less sensitive than primary cell lines for detecting low amount of infectivity. FMDV shows good growth on BHK-21 cell line enabling large-scale production of antigen with good complement fixing properties. The BHK- 21 cell culture provides better growth for FMDV than the suspension culture (Revenson and Segura 1963). The field isolates of FMDV can be passaged in BHK21 clone 13 monolayer cell culture, which showed characteristic CPE and are readily adapted between 3rd and 5th passage (Longjam *et al.*, 2010). The CPE usually develops within 48 hours. If no CPE develops, the cells should be frozen and thawed and are to be inoculated in fresh cultures and examined for CPE for another 48 hours (Goel and Rai 1985). An alternative to the virus isolation is cell suspension plaque test which also quantify the virus present in sample (Barteling *et al.*, 1982). However, the cell culture system is laborious, time consuming and has relatively low sensitivity. It also requires careful handling of specimens and a biosafety laboratory. Further, cell culture loses the sensitivity due to presence of inhibitors like interferons and presence of some enzymatic inhibitors.

4.1.6.2. Complement Fixation Test (CFT)

CFT has been used extensively for distinguishing different strains of FMDV. Subsequently, a modification of CFT known as micro-CFT had been developed wherein 96 well microtiter plates were used instead of tubes (Darbyshire *et al.*, 1972). In the years 1964-1965 CFT tube test was used to replace the virus type identification by guinea pig cross-protection test. Subsequently, the micro-CFT was adopted for this purpose. Although CFT is a fast method it needs high virus load and results are sometimes affected by pro-and anticomplementary activities of the test sample.

4.1.6.3. Neutralization tests

The availability of cell culture techniques and the realization that FMDV can be grown in vitro cultured cells made possible the adaption of neutralization test for routine type identification of FMDV isolates and were found to be more specific than CFT (Rweyemamu 1982). In particular, virus isolation requires a laboratory cell culture facility, which can be difficult and expensive to maintain, besides requiring 4 to 6 days for test completion. Subsequently microneutralization test (MNT) has been used for the assessment of antigenic variation in field strains, as it correlated well with cattle protection test (Rweyemamu 1984). But it has been observed that minimal heterotypic contamination in the sample could interfere with precise type identification of the virus. On the other hand Virus Neutralization test depends on tissue culture and is more prone to variability than ELISA and also require biocontainment facilities.

4.1.6.4. Enzyme linked immuno sorbent assay (ELISA)

A sandwich ELISA using convalescent bovine immunoglobulin as capture and anti-146S guinea pig sera as tracing sera has been found suitable for detection and quantification of FMD virus in infected tissue culture fluid and epithelial tissue samples (Crowther and Elzein 1979). The use of anti-146S rabbit immunoglobulin in place of convalescent bovine immunoglobulin as capture antibody has increased the sensitivity of sandwich ELISA (Ouldridge *et al.*, 1982). Despite being a rapid test, sandwich ELISA has lower analytical sensitivity and is not suitable for use with certain sample types (Hoffmann *et al.*, 2009). Afterwards, ELISA and its various modifications has been applied from time to time for detection, typing, and strain differentiation of FMDV isolates with better sensitivity than CFT and, the results were comparable to that obtained with MNT (Pattnaik and Venkataraman 1989). Liquid phase blocking ELISA (LPBE) using bovine convalescent sera for characterization of field isolates has also been performed and results when tallied with conventional VNT, it is found that ELISA results are much more reproducible than those obtained with VNT and are not influenced by variations in tissue culture susceptibility (Lunt *et al.,* 1994). The Central Laboratory of the Project Directorate at Mukteswar, prepares and optimizes the reagents required both for sandwich ELISA as well as for LPBE. These reagents and other consumables are distributed to the Regional Centres and Network Units on demand. It also repeats the tests, both sandwich ELISA and LPBE on the samples referred to the Central Laboratory by the Regional Centres/Units.

4.1.6.5. Different versions of Polymerase Chain Reaction in FMDV diagnosis

4.1.6.5.1. Reverse Transcription-Polymerase Chain Reaction (rt-PCR)

A specific RT-PCR has been developed and validated for the detection of the polymerase gene (3D) of FMD with an analytical sensitivity 1000 times higher than that of a single passage virus isolation (Moonen *et al.,* 2003). In a study to compare the sensitivity of assays for the diagnosis of FMD, a cell suspension plaque test on BHK21-CT cells and a reverse transcription nested PCR (rt-nPCR) were used to examine nasal swabs and probang samples obtained from FMDV infected cattle, it has been observed that examination of nasal swab revealed a higher number of infected animals using rtnPCR than by the use of the plaque tests and for probing samples both test gave approximately equivalent result (Moss and Haas 1999). PCR products generated have currently only been analyzed by gel electrophoresis exposing to the chance of post-PCR contamination. However PCR offers potential advantages over other conventional tests as the risk of false negative associated with poor sample handling is limited.

4.1.6.5.2. Multiplex polymerase chain reaction (mPCR)

RT-PCR though has paved the way to more sensitive and rapid test in the field of molecular diagnosis, serotyping of FMDV has been difficult and this has been solved with the advent of multiplex PCR (mPCR). To overcome the inherent disadvantage of cost and to improve the diagnostic capacity of the test, multiplex PCR came into play which can amplify more than one target sequence using more than one pair of primers in infected tissues and food samples. An advantage of multiplex PCR systems, compared with probebased assays, is that the intrinsic design does not rely on a probe for a single conserved gene or region of the genome. Rather, the multiplex system is designed to survey multiple regions of the genome simultaneously, thereby increasing the probability of detection. To date, these mPCR assays are limited to partial serotyping of FMDV because no existing multiplex PCR assay offer complete coverage for all seven serotypes (Tam *et al.*, 2009). Multiplex PCR can also be used for the differential diagnosis of various vesicular diseases like Vesicular Stomatitis, Swine Vesicular Disease, Vesicular Exanthema from FMD (Lomakina *et al.*, 2004). Recently, mPCR for differentiation of Indian FMDV serotypes has been developed and evaluated on tongue epithelium and cell culture samples (Giridharan *et al.*, 2001). mPCR is also found to be more efficient in detecting FMDV serotypes compared to sandwich ELISA (Longjam *et al.*, 2012).

4.1.6.5.3. Real time polymerase chain reaction (RT-PCR)

Real-time PCR has engendered wider acceptance of PCR due to its improved rapidity and sensitivity overcoming poor precision, low sensitivity, low resolution, absence of automation, only size-based discrimination, absence of expression of results in numbers, poor quantitative performance and post-PCR processing, proving the conventional PCR not very suitable for accurate diagnosis. There are currently five main chemistries used for the detection of PCR product during real-time PCR. These are the DNA-binding fluorophores, the 5' endonuclease, adjacent linear and hairpin oligoprobes, and the selffluorescing amplicons (Mackay *et al.*, 2002). This approach is a highly sensitive technique enabling simultaneous amplification and quantification of specific nucleic acid sequences. In addition to enhanced sensitivity, the benefits of real-time PCR assays over conventional endpoint detection methods include their large dynamic range, a reduced risk of cross-contamination, an ability to be scaled up for high-throughput applications and the potential for accurate target quantification. Real-time PCR assays recommended by the World Organization for animal health (OIE) for detection of FMDV incorporate universal primers and fluorescent-labeled probes that recognized conserved region within the 5' UTR or conserved gene regions within the RNA-dependent RNA polymerase gene (3Dpol). The use of a specific probe facilitates an increase in specificity compared to conventional agarose-gel-based PCR assays (Callahan *et al.*, 2002).

Recently, TaqMan technology has combined the 5' nuclease activity of the Taq DNA polymerase and forster resonance energy transfer to detect and quantify amplification product in a closed tube format (Kessler *et al.*, 2000). Using this technology real-time PCR has been developed to detect the nucleic acid. This is most sensitive and rapid method to detect the nucleic acid. The viral RNA can be consistently detected over a seven log range, the lowest of which corresponded to as few as 10–100 RNA per volume tested. The test can be performed in 2 hours or less on a portable instrument and sample can be held at ambient temperatures.

4.1.6.6. Recombinant antigen based diagnosis

The 3AB protein of FMDV can be expressed in *E. coli* (Suryanaryana *et al.*, 1999) or in *P. pastoris* and can been used for the diagnosis of FMD infection in cattle. Similarly, 3ABC proteins expressed in heterologous systems can be used in ELISA (3ABC ELISA) for serodiagnosis of FMD (Lu *et al.*, 2007). Further, four serotypes of FMDV structural proteins expressed in *P. pastoris* and its potential utility either as immunogen or antigen has been successfully assessed in animal model (Renji *et al.*, 2003). A recombinant FMDV polyprotein (P1) with 3C expressed in insect cells was evaluated for detecting antibodies to FMDV serotype Asia 1 in ELISA and has the potential to replace the liquid phase blocking (LPB)-ELISA using an inactivated FMDV antigen as a simple and robust serological tool for screening antibodies to FMDV serotype Asia 1 (Ko *et al.*, 2009).

4.1.6.7. Differentiation of infected and vaccinated animals (DIVA) based diagnostic approaches

The ability to identify and selectively delete genes from a pathogen has allowed the development of marker vaccines which when combined with suitable diagnostic assays, allow differentiating infected from vaccinated animals (DIVA) by differentiation of antibody responses induced by the vaccine from those induced during infection with the wild-type virus (Uttenthal *et al.*, 2010). A number of antigenic non-structural proteins (NSPs) of FMD has been identified out of which 3ABC gene appears to be the most reliable marker of FMD virus replication (Henderson 2005). The deletion of NSP (3ABC) gene has been used for enabling DIVA approach for FMD (Cedivac-FMD inactivated vaccine). For detection of NSP antibodies, the Ceditest FMD-NS ELISA is commercially available. Indirect ELISA test for the detection of antibodies against non-structural proteins will play an essential role in the serological survey of livestock herds in future postoutbreak situations. Protection against foot-and-mouth disease (FMD) can be achieved following vaccination with chimera in which the VP1 G-H loop had been substituted with that from another serotype (Fowler *et al.*, 2010). A mutant FMDV with deletion of immuno-dominant epitopes has also been evaluated to use as a marker vaccine in which a B-cell epitope is identified in the 3A region of a nonstructural protein (NSP) by anti-FMDV cattle sera and a recombinant FMDV (rvAs-3A14D) was generated by selectively deleting 14 amino acids (position 91–104) in the 3A region of the NSP. The recombinant FMDV with deletion of this epitope in the

NSP may be potentially used as a candidate inactivated vaccine and therefore, the application of the marker vaccine and differential diagnostic tests may open a promising new avenue for the development of a vaccine for DIVA.

4.1.6.8. Microarray based diagnosis

Microarray-based test that used a FMD DNA chip containing 155 oligonucleotide probes, 35–45 base pairs (bp) long, and serotype-specific, designed from the VP3,VPl-2A region of the genome. A set of two forward primers and one reverse primer have also been designed to allow amplification of approximately 1100 bp of target sequences from this region. The amplified target was labelled with Alexa-Fluor 546 dye and applied to the FMD DNA chip. A total of 23 different FMDV strains representing all seven serotypes were detected and typed by the FMD DNA chip. Microarray technology offers a unique capability to identify multiple pathogens in a single chip (Baxi *et al.*, 2006).

4.1.6.9. Nucleic Acid based approaches

FMDV serotypes A, O, and C was possible, using cDNA probes from individual serotypes that corresponded to structural protein VP1, wherein thirteen complementary DNA (cDNA) probes labelled with 32P has been used to detect the presence of foot-and- mouth disease virus (FMDV) enabled the detection of 1 pg of viral-RNA, or 1 virus copy per cell (McFarlane *et al.*, 1990). A nucleic acid sequence-based amplification (NASBA) assay for the detection of foot-and-mouth disease virus (FMDV) has also been developed (Lau *et al.*, 2008).

4.1.6.10. Phage display based approach

Due to the high antigenic variability of FMDV, it is important to undertake mutation analysis under immunological pressure (Kim *et al.*, 2004). Recently, screening a phage displayed random 12-peptide library, it has been observed that positive phages display the consensus motif ETTXLE (X is any amino acid), which is highly homologous to

6ETTLLE11 at the N-terminus of the structural protein VP2 of FMDV. A minimal epitopic region require to bind a monoclonal antibody of serotype independent FMDV (MAb4B2) and thus can be used as a universal diagnostic candidate.

4.1.6.11. Pen side diagnostic approaches

Development of a rapid chromatographic strip test, the lateral flow device (LFD) for penside diagnosis is based on a monoclonal antibody that reacts against FMDV of all seven serotypes. The lateral flow assay (LFA) permits rapid diagnosis, thus allowing time for the early implementation of control measures to reduce the possibility of spread of FMD. The LFA has been developed widely to support clinical diagnosis of FMD. Again a simple, rapid, colloidal gold-based immuno-chromatographic strip tests is developed for easy clinical testing of serotype A of FMDV in field sites with high sensitivity and specificity (Reid *et al.*, 2001). A new version of loop mediated isothermal amplification (LAMP) called reverse transcription loop mediated isothermal amplification (RT-LAMP) is also developed for rapid, specific and sensitive detection of FMDV in laboratory and in field condition (Dukes *et al.*, 2006).

4.1.7. Prevention and control

Economic consequence is the primary driver of FMD control globally as well as in India. The disease is considered as the number one priority list disease which seeks prevention and control measures. The major measures that are to be undertaken are prior notification to the authority, sero-monitoring of non-vaccinated animals, sero-surveillance of vaccinated animals and restriction over animal movement, both inter-state and trans-boundary. Along with these measures, vaccination coverage is also important.

4.1.7.1. FMD vaccines

All manufacturers use BHK suspension culture technique for manufacture of the oil adjuvated aluminium hydroxide precipitated binaryethyleneimine (BEI) inactivated tissue culture vaccine (Aarthi *et al.,* 2004). Until 2003, FMD vaccine manufacturers in India used different vaccine strains. However, Project Directorate on FMD (PDFMD), ICAR and Govt. of India harmonized the strains used for vaccine production. However, the major shortcoming of such vaccine used for mass vaccination programme is the presence of non-structural protein (NSP). Currently, vaccine manufactured in India varies from NSP free to traces of NSP. It has been observed in the recent past that animal experiments using recombinant FMD NSP antigen and FMD vaccine spiked with native FMD NSP antigen. For proper marketing of vaccines, vaccine manufacturers should undertake validation of inactivation kinetics while introducing new batches of BEI, potency of vaccine should be increased to 6 PD_{50} (still doubtful) and post-marketing surveillance should be made mandatory (Reports of Srinivasan).

Table 8 : Different FMDV serotypes and vaccine strains used for vaccine production

Serotype	Vaccine strain
O	O IND R2/75 from October 2003 onwards
A	A IND 40/00 from September 2008 onwards
Asia 1	Asia 1 IND 63/72 from October 2003 onwards

4.1.7.2. FMD control programmes

Earlier FMD control programmes undertaken in selected districts in southern part of the country could not be sustained. Though vaccination was undertaken during the last 25 years it was not focused till the beginning of the 10th plan (2002-2007). There are two programmes on FMD control presently operational in the country viz., FMD CP (which is 100 per cent Govt. of India funded) and ASCAD programme of Govt. of India and State governments implemented in non FMD states. The experience of the FMDCP has given valuable results so far. It is expected that the programme will be expanded further to cover the entire nation during the 12th plan. The main objective of the programme is repeated mass vaccination of all cattle population of the country and establishment of one or more clearly defined zones to attain 'Freedom with vaccination status' by 2020. Presently, State Governments collect serum samples from vaccinated animals in FMDCP area which are analyzed by the PDFMD laboratories located in different states. The PDFMD and State Governments regularly undertakes disease surveillance through the epidemiological units. At present, there is one central FMD laboratory (PDFMD), located at Mukteshwar, one SAARC FMD centre, 8 regional centres and 15 network units (Reports of Venkataraman).

4.2. Infectious bovine rhinotracheitis and infectious pustular vulvovaginitis (IBR- IPV)

4.2.1. Introduction

Infectious bovine rhinotracheitis/infectious pustular vulvovaginitis (IBR/IPV), caused by bovine herpesvirus 1 (BoHV-1), is a disease of domestic and wild cattle. It is a list B disease of the Office International des Epizooties (OIE). It is one of the most widespread respiratory/reproductive viral diseases of bovines in India (Kiran *et al.* 2005). India has massive cattle and buffalo populations which are frequently exposed to. IBR which has been known to exist in India since 1976 (Mehrotra 1977). The isolation of BHV-1 from the respiratory and genital tracts of bovines has been reported from the states of Orissa, Karnataka and Gujarat. Furthermore, widespread serological evidence of respiratory as well as genital tract infections is reported from most of the states in India (Suribabu *et al.,* 1984). IBR infection assumes great economic importance in India, which is the second largest milk producer in the world. Moreover, the dairy industry is poised for rapid growth with the introduction of exotic germplasm for crossbreeding with the indigenous cattle population. The disease causes abortions, infertility, meningoencephalitis, keratoconjunctivitis, respiratory and genital tract infections.

4.2.2. Etiological agent

BoHV-1 is a member of the genus *Varicellovirus* in the subfamily *Alphaherpesvirinae*, which belongs to the family *Herpesviridae* under the order *Herpesvirales*. The viral genome consists of double-stranded DNA that encodes for about 70 proteins out of which there are 33 structural and more than 15 nonstructural proteins. The viral glycoproteins located in the envelope on the surface of the virion play an important role in pathogenesis and immunity. BoHV-1 can be differentiated into subtypes 1.1, 1.2a and 1.2b (Metzler *et al.*, 1985). The BoHV-1.2 subtypes may be less virulent than subtype 1.1 (Edwards *et al.*, 1990). The former BoHV-1.3, which may act as a neuropathogenic agent in calves, has been reclassified as BoHV-5 (Magyar *et al.*, 1993). BoHV-1 shares antigenic and genetic close relationships with other ruminant alphaherpesviruses *viz.*, BoHV-5, caprine herpesvirus 1, cervid herpesvirus 1 (red deer), cervid herpesvirus 2 (reindeer), bubaline herpesvirus 1 and elk herpesvirus 1 (Thiry *et al.*, 2006).

4.2.3. Virus transmission and pathogenesis

After infection via the airborne route, BoHV-1 replicates to high titres in mucous membranes of the upper respiratory tract and in the tonsils. Subsequently, the virus disseminates to conjunctivae and reaches the trigeminal ganglia by neuronal axonal transport. After genital infection, BoHV-1 replicates in the mucous membranes of the vagina or prepuce and ultimately becomes latent in the sacral ganglia. The viral DNA remains in the neurons of the ganglia, probably for the entire life of the host and assumes the status of latency. Stress, such as transport and parturition, but also the application of corticosteroids can induce reactivation of the latent infection. Consequently, the virus may switch between latent and lytic infection and may be shed intermittently into the environment and spread to contact animals. BoHV-1 infection elicits an antibody response and a cell-mediated immune response within 7–14 days. The immune response is presumed to persist life-long, although it may fall below the detection limit of some tests after a number of years. Maternal antibodies are transferred via colostrum to the young calf, which is consequently protected against BoHV-1-induced clinical disease (Mechor *et al.*, 1987). Maternal antibodies have a biological half-life of about 3 weeks, but may be detected occasionally in animals up to 9 months old, and rarely in animals over this age. The serological presence of IBR with low antibody titres when no clinical history is available could be interpreted as evidence of past infection with IBR virus or as slow antibody response following primary infection (Suresh *et al.*, 1999).

4.2.4. Clinical signs

After an incubation period of 2–4 days, serous nasal discharge, salivation, fever, inappetence, and depression become evident. Within a few days the nasal and ocular discharges change to mucopurulent. Where natural mating is practised, genital infection can lead to pustular vulvovaginitis or balanoposthitis. However, most infections run a very mild or subclinical course (Van Oirschot *et al.*, 1993). Uncomplicated cases of respiratory or genital disease caused by BoHV-1 last for about 5–10 days. Secondary bacterial or viral agents may contribute to a multifactor disease complex resulting in severe respiratory disease of young animals and such form of the disease is known as shipping or crowding fever.

4.2.5. Diagnosis

4.2.5.1. Virus isolation

For virus isolation, bovine cells of various origins can be used. Primary or secondary bovine kidney, lung or testis cells, cell strains derived from bovine fetal lung, turbinate or trachea, and established cell lines like the Madin–Darby bovine kidney cell line (MDBK) are suitable for BoHV-1 propagation. The most suitable sample for virus isolation is the susceptible bull semen which is prescribed for international trade. The CPE is characterised by grapelike clusters of rounded cells gathered around a hole in the monolayer and sometimes giant cells with several nuclei may be observed (Brunner *et al.*, 1988). To identify the recovered virus as BoHV-1, the supernatant of the culture should be neutralised with a monospecific BoHV-1 antiserum or neutralising monoclonal antibody (MAb). An alternative method of virus identification is the direct verification of BoHV-1 antigen in cells around the CPE by an immunofluorescence or immunoperoxidase test (Kaashoek *et al.*, 1994) with conjugated monospecific antiserum or MAb.

4.2.5.2. Immunofluorescence and immunohistochemistry for viral antigen detection

Nasal, ocular, genital swabs and frozen section of tissues collected at post-mortem can be directly smeared onto glass cover-slips, or, following centrifugation, the cell deposit can be spotted onto cover-slips which are subjected to a standard direct or indirect immunofluorescence test. To obtain reliable results, it is necessary to sample several animals in a herd that have fever and a slight, serous nasal discharge. Smears should be air-dried and fixed in acetone. Smears from nasal swabs from cattle with a purulent or haemorrhagic nasal discharge are often negative (Terpstra, 1979). The advantage of this antigen-detection technique is that it can lead to a conclusive diagnosis in a single day. However, the sensitivity of this procedure is lower than that of virus isolation (Edwards *et al.*, 1983) or PCR. Positive and negative controls must be included in each test.

Immunohistochemistry may also be applied for BoHV-1 detection and determination of the antigen location in the tissues. MAbs are increasingly being used for detecting BoHV-1 antigen, leading to enhanced specificity of the test. However, such MAbs must be carefully selected as they must be directed against conserved epitopes that are present on all isolates of BoHV-1.

4.2.5.3. Serological tests

Virus neutralisation (VN) tests and various ELISAs are usually used for detecting antibodies against BoHV-1 in serum. Because virus latency is a normal sequel to BoHV-1 infection, the identification of serologically positive animals provides a useful and reliable indicator of infection status. Any animal with antibodies to the virus is considered to be a carrier and potential intermittent excretor of the virus. The only exceptions are calves that have acquired passive colostral antibodies from their dam, and non-infected cattle vaccinated with inactivated vaccines. There is also a risk that calves infected under cover of maternal immunity may become serologically negative while carrying a reactivatible latent infection (Lemaire *et al.*, 2000).

In general, BoHV-1 serological tests can be divided into conventional and marker tests. Till date, the only serological marker tests available are the BoHV-1 gE-antibody blocking ELISAs (OIE 2010). Animals vaccinated with gE-deleted marker vaccines can be discriminated from field-virus infected animals by a negative serological reaction for gE. The gE-ELISA, are increasingly used for the detection of antibodies in (bulk) milk samples (Wellenberg *et al.*, 1998a), but have some limitations. By testing bulk milk, a positive gB-specific test indicates that the infection has already spread in the herd (Frankena *et al.*, 1997). With the gE-blocking ELISA, bulk milk gives a positive reaction when more than 10–15% of the herd is infected ((Wellenberg *et al.*, 1998b). Consequently, it is not possible to declare a herd to be free from BoHV-1 infection with these tests on the basis of bulk or pooled milk samples, and a negative gE- or gB-ELISA bulk milk test should be followed up with individual blood samples from all cattle in the herd. For conventional serology, VNT, BoHV1-antibody blocking ELISAs and indirect ELISAs may be used. Indirect ELISAs optimised for use with bulk milk samples of up to 50 individual cows can indicate reliably the BoHV-1 status of these animals. For general surveillance purposes, bulk milk tank tests can give an estimate of BoHV-1 prevalence in a herd, an area or country (Nylin *et al.*, 2000). These should be supplemented by serum testing (individual or pooled) from non-milking herds. For monitoring a BoHV-1 status in dairy herds, bulk milk samples of up to 50 animals should be tested 3–4 times per year with a suitable indirect ELISA. Avidin-Biotin ELISA has been specifically developed for the diagnosis of IBR as the technique is highly sensitive, specific and very economical, since it allows the use of immunoconjugates at very high dilution, as compared to indirect ELISA (Babu and Rajasekhar 1988).

Virus neutralization tests (VNTs) are performed with various modifications. Tests vary with regard to the virus strain (Perrin *et al.*, 1993). Various bovine cells or cell lines are suitable for use in the VN test, including secondary bovine kidney or testis cells, cell strains of bovine lung or tracheal cells, or the established Madin–Darby bovine kidney (MDBK) cell line.

4.2.5.4. Molecular diagnostic tools

PCR has been used mainly to detect BoHV-1 DNA in artificially or naturally infected semen samples. The TK, gB, gC, gD and gE genes have been used as targets for PCR amplification. In addition, PCRs based on detection of gE sequences can be used to differentiate between wild-type virus and gE-deleted vaccine strains (Fuchs *et al.*, 1999). Discrimination between infection with virulent IBR strains and infection with live attenuated strains is not possible with the PCR technique, and RFLP is used for this purpose. Specific PCRs have been developed that are able to discriminate between BoHV-1, BoHV-5 and other related alphaherpesviruses (Ros *et al.*, 1999). The major advantage of using PCR is that it is found to be more sensitive than virus isolation. It has been found that in egg yolk-extended semen samples obtained from experimentally infected bulls, PCR can detect five times as many positives as do virus isolation (Van Engelenburg *et al.*, 1995). The detection limit of validated PCR assays amounts to only a few genome copies per PCR reaction. However, the possibility of occurrence of false-negative results cannot be excluded. To identify possible false-negative results, it is recommended to spike an internal control template into the reaction tube of the semen sample to be amplified by the same primers.

The real time (RT) PCR used for detection of BoHV -1 uses a pair of sequence-specific primers for amplification of a 97 base pair sequence of the glycoprotein B (gB) gene (Grom *et al.*, 2006) of all BoHV-1 strains including subtype 1 and 2 from extended bovine semen and a 5'-nuclease oligoprobe for detection of amplified products. The oligoprobe is a single, sequence-specific oligonucleotide, labelled with two different fluorophores, the reporter, 5- carboxyfluorescein (FAM) at the 5' end, and the quencher 6-carboxytetramethylrhodamine (TAMRA) at the 3' end.

4.2.6. Prevention and control

Prevention and control of BoHV-1 infections are based on thorough farm management including hygienic measures, vaccination schedules and removal of infected animals. Ideally, quarantine for 4 weeks period is imposed for newly introduced cattle, if the cattle are not from certified BoHV-1-free farms. Only cattle that are BoHV-1-sero-negative are then admitted to a free herd. Natural mating should be avoided and only semen from BoHV-1- negative bulls should be used. Vaccines usually prevent the development of clinical signs and markedly reduce the shedding of virus after infection, but do not completely prevent infection. Several attenuated and inactivated BoHV-1 vaccines are currently available. The vaccine strains have usually undergone multiple passages in cell culture. Some of the vaccine virus strains have a temperature- sensitive phenotype that do not replicate at temperatures of 39°C or higher. Attenuated vaccines are administered intranasally or intramuscularly. Inactivated vaccines contain high levels of inactivated virus or portions of the viral glycoproteins supplemented with an adjuvant to stimulate an adequate immune response. Inactivated vaccines are given intramuscularly or subcutaneously. DIVA vaccines are now available in various countries. These are attenuated or inactivated marker vaccines which are based on deletion mutants (deletion of gE) or on a subunit of the virion like glycoprotein D. The use of such marker vaccines in conjunction with companion diagnostic tests allows the distinction between infected and vaccinated cattle and provides the basis for BoHV-1 eradication programmes in countries or regions with a high prevalence of field-virus infected animals. Intensive vaccination programmes can reduce the prevalence of infected animals (Mars *et al.*, 2001). Ultimately, vaccination against BoHV-1 is used to protect animals from the clinical outcome of infection, and as an aid in control and eradication programme.

4.3. Rota viral diarrhoea

4.3.1. Introduction

Amongst the various causes of neonatal diarrhoea, group A rotavirus has a world-wide distribution and is considered to be the single most important aetiological agent of acute viral gastroenteritis (Flewett and Woode 1978) various mammalian species including new borne calves and provoke economic losses. Contamination of calves by rotavirus occurs soon after birth. The main source of virus in the surroundings seems to be the faeces of diarrhoeic calves, but it has also been observed with a high frequency in stools of apparently healthy ones (Pastoret *et al.,* 1984).

4.3.2. Etiological agent and its grouping

Rotaviruses have a distinct wheel like appearance by negative–stain electron microscopy (EM) and thus have been named *rota* (in *latin* means wheel). It is a non-enveloped virus of the family Reoviridae having a genome of 11 segments of double-stranded RNA, of molecular weight 2 x 105 to 2.2 x 106 daltons, which is encased within a triple, layered capsid (Ciarlet and Estes 1999), the innermost layer of which, the core, contains the viral genome. Each RNA segment encodes a single viral polypeptide for 6 structural (VP1, VP2, VP3, VP4, VP6, VP7) and 5 non structural proteins (NSP1-NSP5). The structural proteins are located in the core (VP1-VP3), inner shell (VP6) and outershell (VP4, VP7) (Desselberger 1998). The two most important outer capsid proteins are VP4 and VP7, both of which are independently responsible for virus neutralisation (Estes 2001). Antigenic specificity carried by the VP4 and VP7 proteins is termed

P and G genotype or serotype respectively (Estes and Cohen 1989). Rotaviruses are classified into seven groups *viz.*, A to G and several subgroups based on specificity of VP6 inner shell polypeptide. Groups A, B and C are associated with both human and animal infections whereas groups D, E, F and G are associated with diarrhoea in only animals. Group A viruses are mainly associated with diarrhoea in calves and are further classified into subgroups I, II, I+II and non I and II according to exclusive reactivities of two VP6-specific monoclonal antibodies. Types within group A are determined by cross-neutralization studies as serotypes or by sequence comparison as genotype. The VP4 and VP7 outer capsid proteins independentently induces antibodies associated with type specific neutralization and protection from infection. However, the strains of rota virus are further classified into electropherotypes on the basis of differences in the relative migration rates of genome segments in polyacrylamide gel electrophoresis (PAGE), creating more opportunity for strain diversification (Kapikian *et al.,* 2001). Till date, group A rotaviruses have been characterised as possessing 15 G and 21 P genotypes (Das *et al.,* 2002). To establish preventive measures against diarrhoea caused by group A rotaviruses, G and P type bovine rotavirus (BRV) distribution has been frequently investigated throughout the world (Fukai *et al.,* 2002). At least nine G types (G1-G4, G6-G8, G10 and G11) have been identified in bovine group A rotavirus strains (Okada and Matsumoto 2002). According to previous reports, G6 and G10 have been identified as the most common G types of BRV. In India, although the occurrence of BRV-related diarrhoea has been well documented, only one report is available on the distribution of G and P types (Gulati *et al.,* 1999). Nevertheless, it is proven that co-circulation of diverse strains of *Rotavirus* in a particular area may be due to either the existence of diverse strains or emergence of variation

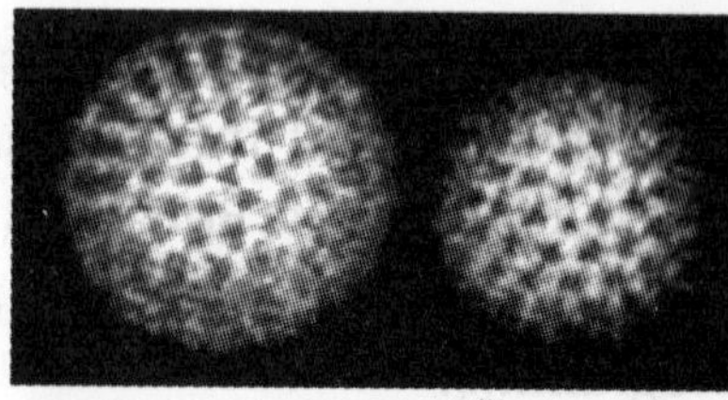

Fig. 19 : Rota virus. A double-capsid particle (left) and a single, inner capsid (right) (http://www.pathomicro.med.sc.edu).

in the electropherotypes by natural reassortment between two strains of *Rotavirus* (Gulati *et al.*, 1995).

4.3.3. Sources and transmission of infection

Rotavirus does not seem to cross the placental barrier (Dagenais *et al.*, 1980a). This is not surprising since there is still no definite evidence of occurance of viraemia after rotavirus infection (Vanden Broecke *et al.*, 1984a) and specific anti-rotavirus antibodies have never been detected in pre-colostral calf sera (Dagenais *et al.*, 1981), although the bovine foetus is perfectly able to produce an immune response against rotavirus antigens from the 127th day of its development (Schlaffer *et al.*, 1979). Contamination of newborn calves occurs, therefore, very soon after birth, as in natural conditions rotavirus excretion has been observed within 48 hours after birth (Mc Nulty *et al.*, 1976). Asymptomatic excretion of rotavirus by adult cows is uncommon and therefore does not seem to play a significant role in the dissemination of the virus (Dagenais *et al.*, 1980b). The main source of rotavirus in the surroundings seems to be the faeces of diarrhoeic calves that contain large amounts of viral particles (Van Opdenbosch *et al.*, 1979). Nevertheless, rotavirus has also been observed in the stools of apparently healthy calves (Scherrer *et al.*, 1976). This may be due either to prolonged asymptomatic viral multiplication, or due to successive re-infections. The second hypothesis is the more likely one as re-infection of dogs, cats or calves leads to re-excretion of rota virus (Schwers *et al.*, 1984). Moreover, rotavirus is highly resistant and contamination through humans, contaminated material or infected areas certainly plays a role in the transmission of the infection (Woode 1978). Moreover, rotavirus, most probably of bovine origin has been isolated from stools of farm dogs (Hoyois *et al.*, 1982), showing that cross-contamination occurs in normal breeding conditions. Because of their presence in most of the farms, often in close contact with calves, dogs and cats may play a role in the maintenance of rota virus infection (Schwers *et al.*, 1983).

4.3.4. Factors affecting the pathogenicity of bovine rota virus

The dose of the virus is an important factor controlling the occurrence of diarrhoea in calves. Interestingly, very high dose of cell culture derived bovine rota virus fails to reproduce diarrhoea in colostrums deprived new borne calves whereas lower doses succed because of the phenomen of interference (Vanden Broecke *et al.*, 1984b). The age of the animal at the time of infection may play a crucial role as the susceptibility to rota virus infections in new born calves decreases as the animal becomes older (Snodgrass *et al.*, 1976). Generally, a protease is required to remove some of the outer layer of the capsid and to generate an intermediate sub-viral particle (ISVP) before the virus can enter the cytoplasm. *In vivo*, the ISVPs are probably generated by protease digestion in the GI tract. A viral attachment protein is then exposed on the ISVP, probably at the vertices, and binds to host cell receptors. Ingestion of excessive quantity of milk may activate the lactate dehydrogenase enzyme that promotes the ISVP formation by cleaving the outer capsid proteins of the virus, thereby facilitating the invasion of the intestinal epithelial cells by the sub-viral agents. Differences also exist between virus isolates in their ability to affect animals of different ages (Bridger 1980). The role of concomitant infections by other viruses, bacteria or other infectious agents must also be taken into consideration. For example, it is well known that the association between rotavirus and enteropathogenic *E. coli* increases the pathogenicity of both agents (Tzipori *et al.*, 1981).

4.3.5. Diagnosis

Rotavirus is excreted in large numbers in the faeces (>106 particles/g faeces) and thus can be easily identified on electron microscopy of stool samples and it is one of the most specific tests for diagnosis (Kapikian *et al.*, 1976.). Direct EM examination of stools for rotavirus has a sensitivity of 80-90 per cent. However EM requires expensive equipment and trained personnel and thus cannot be used in field studies. Virus isolation can be performed in intestinal cells of bovine origin wit the addition of trypsin (as trypsin facilitates the formation of ISVP formation). Other methods like immunoelectro-osmophoresis and modified complement fixation test have also been developed, but they lack sensitivity. Following this, many rapid and economical assays like latex agglutination (LA), reverse passive haemagglutination assay (RPHA), solid phase agglutination of coated erythrocytes (SPACE), enzyme immuno assay (EIA) and poly-acrylamide gel electrophoresis (PAGE) have been used from time to time for diagnosis (Singh *et al.*, 1986; Dar *et al.*, 1994). However, the most widely used methods currently are Latex agglutination (LA), ELISA and RNA-PAGE. ELISA using polyclonal sera may give false positive results and requires validation by confirmatory or blocking ELISA (Cukor and Blacklow 1984). However, specific ELISA assays based on monoclonal antibodies (Coulson *et al.*, 1999) and polyclonal antibody based sandwich ELISA have been developed for identifying the genomic diversity and prevalence of rota virus (Jindal *et al.*, 2000). RNA-PAGE followed by silver staining is a primary identifier of different strains (electropherotypes) of rota virus in faeces of diarrhoeic calves and is a highly specific technique (Dash *et al.*, 2011) to obtain important epidemiological data on rotavirus disease outbreaks but it lacks sensitivity as a minimum of 3-4ng of viral RNA is needed for detection (Herring *et al.*, 1981). New methods like dot blot hybridization using radio labelled cDNA probes and reverse transcriptase– polymerase chain reaction (RT-PCR) are now being used as confirmatory methods for detecting rotavirus in faecal samples. RT-PCR has been found to be a highly sensitive and specific method for diagnosis of rotavirus in stool sample from patients with acute diarrhoea (Husain *et al.*, 1995).

4.3.6. Prevention in the limelight of control of virus multiplication in calves

The presence of circulating anti-rotavirus antibodies of colostral origin does not prevent rota virus diarrhoea in new born calves. To protect the animal, antibodies must be present in the intestinal lumen (Snodgrass and Wells 1978). This is not surprising since rota virus multiplies only in the epithelial cells of the gut (Mc Nulty 1978), and, therefore, escapes contact with circulating antibodies, which are thus unable to neutralize it. Actively acquired immunity, as demonstrated by seroconversion, is also not sufficient to protect calves againts reinfections. The percentage of animals possessing anti- rota virus antibodies in a herd is an epidemiological indicator, depending upon management conditions, but is not directly related to the prevalence of calf diarrhoea in the farm. A mechanism susceptible of playing an important role in the control of rotavirus multiplication is the endogenous interferon response. Bovine rota virus seems to be very susceptible to interferon. New born calves experimentally infected with bovine rota virus produce high levels of interferon in the lumen of the gut but also in their plasma (La Bonnardiere 1981). Because of the susceptibility of the bovine rota virus to interferon, exogenous bovine or simian interferons or inducers of endogenous interferons can be given to new born calves to prevent the onset of diarrhoea (Werenne 1982). Attempts to vaccinate have often been unsuccessful (Flewett and Woode 1978). However, cows respond heterotypically after monovalent vaccination to all rotavirus serotypes with which they have had experience and, therefore, that single serotype vaccination may be sufficient (Snodgrass *et al.,* 1984).

Moreover, calves suffer from repeated infections after birth. Better results can be obtained by prolonged administration of colostrum to calves, usually associated with vaccination of cows to obtain higher antibody levels in the colostrum and milk (Van Opdenbosch 1982). Among the drugs, bismuth subsalicylate may be useful as it has been shown to inhibit the multiplication of bovine rota virus in cell cultures and also to absorb the enterotoxin produced by enteropathogenic strains of *Escherichia coli* (Josse *et al.,* 1979).

4.4. Rabies

4.4.1. Introduction

Rabies is an acute viral encephalomyelitis that may affect all warm blooded animals including cattle. The disease is an acute, progressive encephalitis caused by a lyssavirus. Rabies virus is the most important lyssavirus globally (Blanton *et al.*, 2010) as well as in India. The infection creates a progressive inflammation of the brain. Inlarge parts of the world, dogs are the main source of infection to other animals. Endemic or sporadic rabies in wild life or stray animals can easily spill over to domestic cattle. It is a notifiable disease in the OIE list.

4.4.2. Etiological agent

As mentioned earlier, rabies is caused by the bullet shaped lyssa virus under the family *Rhabdoviridae*. Eleven distinct species have been identified within the genus, namely classical rabies virus (RABV), Lagos bat virus (LBV), Mokola virus (MOKV), Duvenhage virus (DUVV), European bat lyssaviruses type-1 (EBLV1) and type-2 (EBLV2), Australian bat lyssavirus (ABLV) and four lyssaviruses (Aravan virus (ARAV), Khujand virus (KHUV), Irkut virus (IRKV) and West Caucasian bat virus (WCBV). However, in India, the disease causing agent is mainly RABV. All lyssaviruses tested till date cause clinical disease indistinguishable from classical rabies. Conserved antigenic sites on the nucleocapsid proteins permit recognition of all lyssaviruses with modern commercial preparations of anti-rabies antibody conjugates used for diagnostic tests on brain tissue. The Lyssaviruses have been divided into two phylogroups with distinct pathogenicity and immunogenicity (Badrane *et al.*, 2001). For RABV, conserved antigenic sites on the surface glycoproteins allow cross-neutralisation and cross-protective immunity to be elicited by rabies vaccination.

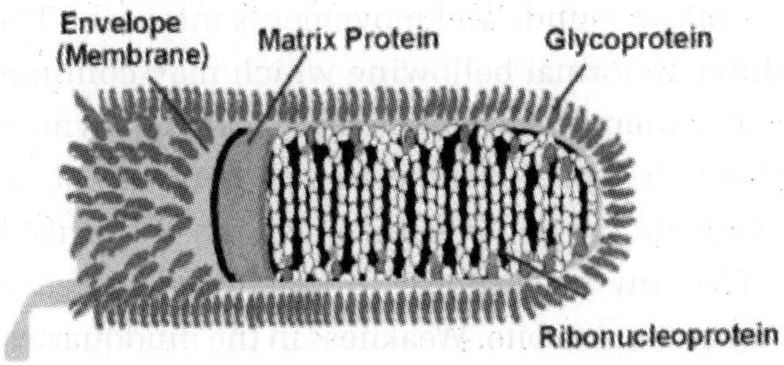

Fig. 20 : Bullet shaped Rabies virus in its simplest form (http://www.microbeworld.org)

4.4.3. Transmission, pathogenesis and shedding

Transmission is usually by the introduction of virus-laden saliva into the tissues of a cow by the bite of a rabid animal. In cattle, the incubation period is usually about 3 weeks, but may be anywhere from 2 weeks to several months in length and often depends on the area where the animal was bitten and the amount of virus present in the bite. Following entry, during the incubation period, the virus initially multiplies in myocytes, enters the nerve endings and subsequently axon cytoplasm and spinal cord and ultimately affects the brain. This is known as the centripetal migration. In brain, virus multiplies predominantly in the nerve cells that drives the animal into frenzies of rage. Multiplication in brain gives rise to the typical intracytoplasmic inclusion bodies called the negri bodies. This is followed by centrifugal migration of the virus through efferent system and dissemination in the salivary glands, peripheral nerve endings and body secretions and excretions. Salivary excretion is very high and intermittent. The disease is generally communicable during the salivary excretion of the virus (Catherine 2011).

4.4.4. Clinical signs

Clinical signs of rabies may vary. The most reliable clinical signs are a sudden change in behavior, unexplained clinical signs that are related to the central nervous system, or progressive paralysis in the affected patient. Two forms of rabies are possible with totally different clinical signs (Bradford 1996). In the furious form of rabies in cattle, normally docile animals may attack humans and other animals. Milk production ceases abruptly in dairy cattle. The cow may appear hypersensitive and will follow sounds and movements intensely. The affected cattle may exhibit abnormal bellowing which may continue intermittently, or voiceless attempts to bellow, the so called yawning. In the paralytic form, the first sign of trouble may be paralysis of the throat. Drooling of saliva, grinding of the teeth, extension of the head, and bloat may occur. The cow may appear to be choked. Animals affected in this way rarely attempt to bite. Weakness in the hindquarters may occur and is always accompanied by decreased sensation to the affected area. Paralysis of the anus and penis in the bull may be seen. Eventually the animal will go down and will be unable to get up as paralysis becomes complete.

4.4.5. Diagnosis

4.4.5.1. Collection and handling of samples

Usually the brain is collected following the opening of the skull and the parts to be collected are preferably Ammon's horn, thalamus, cerebral cortex and medulla oblongata. But in the field or when sampling for large epidemiological studies, such approach may be impractical. In such cases, without opening the skull, there are two approaches for collecting sample viz., occipital foramen route (Barrat and Blancou 1988) and retro-orbital route (Montano Hirose *et al.*, 1991) respectively for brain sampling.

Infectivity at room temperature may be extended for several days if brain material is kept in a mixture of 50% glycerol in phosphate buffered saline (PBS). Glycerol/PBS slows bacterial action and therefore protects against the chemical and biological effects of putrefaction. It does not protect against titre decline due to thermal conditions and therefore, rabies virus being thermo-labile, the virus titre will decline during glycerol/PBS storage. Under normal transport conditions in the Indian condition, this protection may be effective for several days. Thus, whenever possible samples in glycerol/PBS should be kept refrigerated. As the virus is not inactivated by glycerol/PBS, all laboratory tests can be used on these samples.

4.4.5.2. Fluorescent antibody test (FAT)

Because of the less sensitivity, high cost and greater time consumption of the negri body detection technique by Mann's or Sellers staining, the most widely used test as per the recommendation of both WHO and OIE for the diagnosis of rabies is now FAT. This 'gold-standard' test may be used directly on a smear and can also be used to confirm the presence of rabies antigen in cell culture or in brain tissue of mice that have been inoculated for diagnosis. The FAT gives reliable results on fresh specimens within a few hours in more 99% of cases. The FAT is sensitive, specific and cheap. The sensitivity of the FAT depends on the specimen, their degree of autolysis, how comprehensively the brain is sampled and even on the type of lyssavirus.

4.4.5.3. Immunoperoxidase test

Immunoperoxidase methods can be used as an alternative to FAT with the same sensitivity (Lembo *et al.*, 2006), but care should be taken to avoid the risk of nonspecific false-positive results. One added advantage is that peroxidase conjugate may also be used on fresh brain tissue or sections of formalin-fixed tissue for immunohistochemical tests.

4.4.5.4. ELISA and Rapid Immunodiagnostic Test (RIDT)

ELISA for detecting rabies antigen is a variation of the immunochemical test. It is useful for large epidemiological surveys (Xu *et al.*, 2007). The specificity and sensitivity of such tests for locally predominant virus variants should be checked before use. In case of human contact these tests should be used in combination with confirmatory tests such as FAT or virus isolation which will be discussed under the next sub heading.

A rapid immunodiagnostic test (RIDT), developed by Kang *et al.* (2007) is a simple test that can be used under field conditions and in developing countries with limited diagnostic resources.

4.4.5.5. Cell culture

Neuroblastoma cells e.g. N2a, CCL-131 in the American Type Culture Collection (ATCC) are highly susceptible to infection with lyssaviruses. Baby hamster kidney (BHK-21) cells are also sensitive to most street virus isolates without any adaptation step, but should be checked for susceptibility to locally predominant virus variants before use. Cell culture tests may be undertaken in multi-well plastic plates, muli-chambered glass slides or on glass cover-slips. The use of one 4-day passage in four wells of a 96-well microtitre plate has been shown to have satisfactory sensitivity for rabies strains (Rudd & Trimarchi, 1989). Cytotoxicity is a commonly reported factor limiting test robustness. Addition of antibiotics, reduction of the time before changing media to as short as 35 minutes and dilution of samples can reduce the cytotoxicity.

4.4.5.6. Molecular techniques

Various molecular diagnostic tests *viz.*, detection of viral RNA by reverse transcription PCR (RT-PCR), PCR-ELISA, hybridisation *in situ* and real-time PCR are used as rapid and sensitive additional techniques for rabies diagnosis (Fooks *et al.*, 2009). The principle of lyssavirus-specific PCRs is a reverse transcription of the parts of the N gene into complementary DNA followed by the amplification of the cDNA by PCR. Although those molecular tests have the highest level of sensitivity, their use is currently not recommended for routine post-mortem diagnosis of rabies (WHO Expert Committee on Rabies 2005) due to high levels of false positive or false negative results without standardisation and very stringent quality control. But they are useful for confirmatory diagnosis, as a first step in virus typing.

4.4.5.7. Use of serological tests for measurement of adaptive immune response

As neutralising antibodies are considered as key component of the adaptive immune response against rabies virus (Hooper *et al.*, 1998) the gold standard test for detection and measurement of adaptive immune response is virus neutralisation (VN) test. However, indirect ELISAs have been developed that do not require high-containment facilities and produce rapid results. Care should be taken when correlating results between virus neutralisation tests and ELISAs owing to the inherent differences between them. Variable sensitivity and specificity for ELISAs in cattle do exist. Although VN tests are recommended where specific assessment of protection is required, both tests are useful for detecting responses to vaccination if appropriate cut-offs are used. Poor quality sera can cause cytotoxicity in VN tests, which could lead to falsepositive results. For such samples, the use of an indirect ELISA has been shown to be as sensitive and specific as the VN test (Servat *et al.*, 2007).

4.4.6. Prevention and control

The first and foremost part of rabies control programme is defining case by identifying the rabid animal after diagnosis by a qualified laboratory. The national case definition for animal rabies requires laboratory confirmation by either a positive direct fluorescent antibody test or isolation of rabies virus in cell culture (Council of State and Territorial Epidemiologists 2009).

Enhanced laboratory-based rabies surveillance and variant typing are essential components of rabies prevention and control programs. Accurate and timely information and reporting is necessary to determine the management of potentially exposed animals, to aid in emerging pathogen discovery, to describe the epidemiology of the disease and to assess the need for and effectiveness of vaccination programs for domestic animals and wildlife. Every animal submitted for rabies testing should be reported for evaluating surveillance trends. Electronic laboratory reporting and notification of animal rabies surveillance data should be implemented. Optimal information on animals submitted for rabies testing should include point location, vaccination history, rabies virus variant (if rabid) and exposures to rabid animals. Integration with standard public health reporting and notification systems is also necessary in this regard (Blanton *et al.*, 2009).

Animal rabies vaccination and exposure histories often are not available for displaced animals. Disaster response creates situations where animal caretakers might lack appropriate training and preexposure vaccination. In such situations, it is critical to implement and co-ordinate rabies prevention and control measures to reduce the risk of rabies transmission and the need for human PEP. Such measures include actions to coordinate relief efforts of individuals and organizations with the local emergency operations center before deployment, to examine each animal at a triage site for possible bite injuries or signs of rabies, isolating animals exhibiting signs of rabies, ensuring that all animals have a unique identifier, administering a rabies vaccination to all animals in the shed unless a reliable proof of vaccination is obtained, adopting minimal standards for animal caretakers as feasible, including personal protective equipments, pre-exposure rabies vaccination, appropriate training in animal handling, providing facilities to confine and observe animals involved in exposure and reporting human exposure to public health authorities. Cattle exposed to a rabid animal and currently vaccinated with a vaccine approved by USDA for that species should be revaccinated immediately and observed for 45 days. However, unvaccinated animal exposed to rabid animal should be euthanized immediately or if it is not feasible due to ethical issues, it should be kept under observation and confined on a case-by-case basis for 6 months (National animal control association guidelines).

Handling and consumption of tissues from exposed animals might carry a risk for rabies transmission. Risk factors depend partially on the site of exposure, amount of virus present, severity of wounds and whether sufficient contaminated tissue has been excised. If an exposed animal is to be custom or home-slaughtered for consumption, it should be done immediately after exposure, and all tissues should be cooked thoroughly. Persons handling exposed animals, carcasses, and tissues should use barrier precautions (Weirtheim *et al.*, 2009). Historically, federal guidelines for meat inspectors required that any animal known to have been exposed to rabies within 8 months be rejected for slaughter (Ante-mortem inspection. *In:* U.S. Meat and poultry inspection program 1973).

4.4.6.1. Vaccines and pre-exposure vaccination

Multiple vaccines are licensed for use in domestic animal species. Vaccines available include inactivated or modified live virus vectored products, products for intramuscular and subcutaneous administration, products with durations of immunity from one to 4 years and products with varying minimum age of vaccination. In market, products like IMRAB are available for pre-exposure vaccination of cattle at 3 months of age and then annually either through intramuscular or subcutaneous route. Vaccinia rabies recombinant-glycoprotein based vaccines has also proved to be effective (Brochier *et al.,* 1991). The rabies-glycoprotein recombinant vaccines are not live rabies vaccines. They are prepared by inserting non-infectious rabies nucleic acid into a vector such as vaccinia or canary pox.

4.5. Blue tongue

4.5.1. Introduction

Bluetongue is an insect-borne viral disease of ruminants. The blue tongue virus is a member of the genus Orbivirus under the *family* Reoviridae. Even though the clinical disease is predominant in sheep, but the disease may cause inapparent infection in cattle. Most importantly, blue tongue virus antibodies have been detected from time to time in cattle in different states of India (Prasad *et al.,* 1992).

4.5.2. Etiological agent, its genomic organization and serotypes predominant in cattle in India

The BT virus (BTV) is the prototype species of the genus *Orbivirus,* family *Reoviridae* and occurs almost globally between latitudes 35° S and 50° N. The BT viral genome comprises 10 double-stranded (ds) RNA segments varying in size from 0.5 to 2.7 kDa encoding seven structural proteins (VP1–VP7) and four non-structural proteins (NS1–NS3 and NS3A) (Roy *et al.,* 1990). The non-structural proteins NS3 and NS3A are encoded by genes inside the 822 nucleotides length segment S10 via two inframe initiation codons. NS3 corresponds to a 229 aminoacid protein with initiation codon nucleotides at the 20–22 nucleotide position. NS3A is a 216 aminoacid protein in which synthesis is initiated by an in-frame downstream AUG codon located at the 59–61 nucleotide position (Roy 1992). These proteins facilitate the egress of virus particles from the infected cells (Han and Harty 2004). The phylogenetic study of S10 and of its constituent protein sequence has enabled the identification of three different genetic groups within BTV which represent monophyletic geographical clusters irrespective of serotype (Bonneau *et al.*, 1999). S10 segment can be of value for developing refined molecular diagnostic methods for BT. The genetic variability of the NS3/NS3A sequence in field strains is likely the consequence of genetic drift with the co-circulation of related genetic variants in vector insects (Bonneau *et al.*, 2001). The apparent conservation of NS3/NS3A amongst different BTV serotypes and strains likely reflects functional constraints on the protein tolerating little variation.

The earliest evidence of BTV infection in bovines in India is documented in the Annual Report of the Indian Veterinary Research Institute (Anon 1978). According to this report, 3.7% of cattle sera were positive for BTV antibodies as detected by the agar gel immunodiffusion (AGID) test. Serological survey conducted in cattle in Punjab revealed the presence of BTV antibodies in 6.8% of cattle sera (Sharma *et al.*, 1985). Cattle sera from seven states *viz.*, Andhra Pradesh, Karnataka, Gujarat, Punjab, Orissa, Himachal Pradesh and West Bengal revealed 18% seropositivity for BTV antibodies (Mehrotra and Shukla 1984). In 1990, an extensive survey of BTV antibodies in cattle was conducted in Haryana and the study revealed 6.9% seropositivity for BTV antibodies in bull sera (Gupta *et al.*, 1990). It has been observed that serotype 1, 3 and 4 are frequently revealed in case of cattle. However, no attempts have been made to date to isolate BTV from semen. No studies have been conducted on the semen quality of bulls with BTV or BTV antibodies. These animals may play an important role in the maintenance of the virus in nature. The presence of BTV antibodies in cattle has become a serious impediment to the export of the germplasm of these animals.

4.5.3. Epidemiology

Bluetongue virus is transmitted by biting midges in the genus *Culicoides* spp. These insect vectors pick up the infection by feeding on viraemic animals. Replication period in the insect's salivary gland is about 6-8 days and such infected midges remain infective for life. The infection progresses in cattle-midges cycle and once a certain level of infection is attained the infection spills over to the significient species of the disease, sheep. Transovarial transmission does not take place in midges. Overwintering of BTV is due to survival of infected midges as well as latently infected cattle.

The prevalence of the disease is governed by ecological factors like high rainfall, temperature and humidity. The climate in India varies quite widely between different parts of the country. The monsoon season lasting from June to October is the most favourable period for multiplication of *Culicoides* spp. During this period, the maximum temperature ranges between 26°C and 40.3° C, relative humidity between 61 % and 8 9% and monthly rainfall between 5.3 and 204 mm. Most of the outbreaks of BT have been recorded in India during this period (Mahajan *et al.*, 1991).

4.5.4. Clinical signs

Infected animal mainly suffers from inapparent infection. Most often, the only signs of disease are changes in the leukocyte count and a fluctuation in rectal temperature. Rarely, animals may have mild hyperemia, vesicles or ulcers in the mouth, hyperemia around the coronary band, hyperesthesia, or a vesicular and ulcerative dermatitis. The skin may develop thick folds, particularly in the cervical region. The external nares may contain erosions and a crusty exudate. Temporary sterility may be seen in bulls. Infected cows can give birth to calves with hydranencephaly or cerebral cysts. Cattle that have clinically apparent disease may develop severe breaks in the hooves several weeks after infection. Such breaks are usually followed by foot rot.

4.5.5. Diagnosis

Bluetongue should be suspected when typical clinical signs are seen during seasons when insects are active. A recent history of wasting and foot rot in the herd supports the diagnosis. The disease should be differentiated from FMD. Blood samples for virus isolation and serum should be collected from several live febrile animals in the early stage of infection. The blood should be collected into a suitable anticoagulant like EDTA or citrate.

4.5.5.1. Virus isolation

Bluetongue can be diagnosed by isolating the virus in embryonated chicken eggs or cell cultures. Appropriate cell cultures include mouse L, baby hamster kidney (BHK)-21, African green monkey kidney (Vero), and *Aedes albopictus* (AA) cells. Isolation in embryonated eggs is more sensitive than isolation in cell culture (Mc Phee *et al.*, 1982).

4.5.5.2. Animal innoculation

Bluetongue virus can also be isolated by inoculation suckling mice or hamsters. Animal inoculation is more sensitive than virus isolation in cell culture, and may be particularly valuable when the virus titer is very low.

4.5.5.3. Serological tests

Bluetongue viruses can be identified to the serogroup level by immunofluorescence, antigen-capture enzyme-linked immunosorbent assay (ELISA) or the Immunospot test and can be serotyped by virus neutralization test. The AGID and indirect ELISA tests can identify serogroup-specific antibodies. The agar gel precipitation test (AGPT) remains one of the most widely-used serological tools for surveys of BTV antibodies (Pearson and Jochim 1979). In India, most of the serological studies have been conducted using AGPT. However, dot immunobinding assay (DIA), a modified enzyme-linked immunosorbent assay (ELISA) on nitrocellulose paper strip, is as sensitive as ELISA and more sensitive than AGPT for serodiagnosis of BTV (Chander *et al.*, 1991).

4.5.5.4. Molecular tools

Molecular beacon (MB) fluorescent probe assays and quantitative real time reverse trasnscriptase (rt) PCR assays are used for rapid detection and quantitation of BTV. The real time rt-PCR detected 103 molecules/PCR reaction and recognises all 10 serotypes studied (BTV-1–BTV-9 and BTV-16) and correctly differentiate between infected and non-infected animals irrespective of the type of sample used (whether blood, organs or cell cultures) (Orru *et al.*, 2006). The MBs are hairpin-shaped oligonucleotide probes, and have the property of fluorescing upon hybridization with a specific target sequence. Their hairpin shape increases target specificity providing a lower background signal compared to that found in other linear probes (Tyagi *et al.*, 1998).

4.5.6. Prevention and control

Disinfectants cannot prevent the transmission of virus between animals. However, where disinfection is warranted, sodium hypochlorite or 3% sodium hydroxide can be used. Insect control is important in limiting the spread of the disease. Synthetic pyrethroids or organophosphates are effective against *Culicoides* spp. Moving animals into barns in the evening can also reduce the risk of infection.

In India, inactivated vaccines are in experimental stages and are expected to be on the market shortly. Inactivated vaccines generate serotype-specific long-lasting protective immunity after two injections and may help in controlling epidemics. Differentiating infected from vaccinated animals (DIVA) is theoretically possible with inactivated vaccines but has not yet been developed, whereas the attenuated live vaccines are not candidates for DIVA. Attenuated live vaccines are efficacious but safety issues are of great concern. New-generation vaccines like subunit vaccines, virus-like particles, core-like particles and vectored vaccines can be employed for DIVA. Recombinant vaccines generate cross-protection against multiple BTV serotypes and have great potential in BT vaccine regimens. Moreover, new-generation vaccines are safe and efficacious experimentally, but large-scale field trials are required in this regard. Alternative areas, such as antivirals, siRNA, interferon and nanotechnology may be of future use in the control of BT (Bhanuprakash *et al.*, 2009).

References

1. Astudillo, V. M. and Rosenberg, F. J. (1983). Relationships between animal viral diseases and socio-economic development. *Rev. sci. tech. Off. Int. Epiz.*, 2(4): 1013-1036.

2. Banerjee, K. (1996). Emerging viral infections with special reference to India. *Ind. J. Med. Res.*, 103: 177-200.

3. Brooksby, J. B. (1982). Portraits of viruses: foot-and-mouth disease virus. *Intervirol.*, 18(1-2): 1–23.

4. Woodbury, E. L. (1995). A review of the possible mechanisms for the persistence of foot-and-mouth disease virus. *Epidemiol. Infect.*, 114(1): 1–13.

5. Tamilselvan, R. P., Dey Sanyal, A. and Pattnaik, B. (2009). Genetic transitions of Indian serotype O Foot and Mouth Disease Virus isolates responsible for field outbreaks during 2001– 2009: a brief note: OIE/FAO Reference laboratories network meeting: New Delhi, India, pp. 11-13.

6. Longjam, N., Deb, R., Sarmah, A. K., Tayo, T., Awachat, V. B. and Saxena, V. K. (2011). A brief revie on the diagnosis of Foot-and-Mouth disease of livestock: Conventional to molecular tools. *Vet. Med. Int.*, volume 2011: 905768. doi: 10.4061/2011/905768.

7. Racaniello, V. R. (2001). Picornaviridae: the viruses and their replication. in *Fields Virol.*, pp. 685–722, Lippincott Williams &Wilkins, Philadelphia, Pa, USA, 3rd edition.

8. Pereira, H. G. (1977). Subtyping of foot-and-mouth disease virus. *Develop. Biol. Standard.*, 35:167– 174.

9. Bandyopadhyay, S. K. Foot and Mouth Disease research in India. PD_FMD.

10. Ahuja, K. L., Kumar, A. and Prasad, S. (1996). Incidence and distribution of foot-andmouth disease virus types in North- West India (1991–93). *Ind. J. Virol.*, 12: 125–127.

11. Sarma, D. K., Dutta, P. K. and Harzarika, A. K. (1992). Foot-andmouth disease in North Eastern India during 1991. *Virus Information Exchange Newsletter for South East Asia and the Western Pacific.*, 9: 63–64.

12. Bachrach, H. L. (1968). Foot-and-mouth disease. *Annu. Rev. Microbiol.*, 22: 201–244.

13. Acharya, R., Fry, E., Stuart, D., Fox, G., Rowlands, D. and Brown, F. (1989). The three-dimensional structure of foot-andmouth disease virus at 2.9 A? resolution. *Nature.*, 337(6209): 709–716.

14. Strohmaier, K., Franze, R. and Adam, K. H. (1982). Location and characterization of the antigenic portion of the FMDV immunizing protein. *J. Gen. Virol.*, 59(2): 295–306.

15. Mason, P. W., Bezborodova, S. V. and Henry, T. M. (2002). Identification and characterization of a cis-acting replication element (cre) adjacent to the internal ribosome entry site of foot-and-mouth disease virus. *J. Virol.*, 76(19): 9686–9694.

16. Grubman, M. J. and Baxt, B. (2004). Foot-and-Mouth Disease. *Clin. Microbiol. Rev.*, 17(2): 465–493.

17. Lopez de Quinto, S., S´aiz, M., de La Morena, D., Sobrino, F. and Mart´ýnez-Salas, E. (2002). IRES-driven translation is stimulated separately by the FMDV 3' NCR and poly(A) sequences. *Nucleic Acids Res.*, 30(20): 4398–4405.

18. Ryan, M. D., King, A. M. Q. and Thomas, G. P. (1991). Cleavage of foot-and-mouth disease virus polyprotein is mediated by residues located within a 19 amino acid sequence. *J. Gen. Virol.*, 72(11): 2727–2732.

19. http://www.els.net.

20. http://www.foot-and-mouth.org.

21. Sellers, R. F. (1971). Quantitative aspects of the spread of foot and mouth disease. *Veterinarian.*, 41: 431–439.

22. Donaldson, A. I., Gibson, C. F., Oliver, R., Hamblin, C. and Kitching, R. P. (1987). Infection of cattle by airborne foot-and-mouth disease virus: minimal doses with O1 and SAT2 strains. *Res. Vet. Sci.*, 43(3): 339–346.

23. Nishiura, H. and Omori, R. (2010). An epidemiological analysis of the foot-and-mouth disease epidemic in Miyazaki, Japan, 2010. *Transboundary and Emerging Dis.*, 57(6): 396–403.

24. Ferguson, N. M., Donnelly, C. A. and Anderson, R. M. (2001). The foot-and-mouth epidemic in Great Britain: pattern of spread and impact of interventions. *Sci.*, 292(5519): 1155–1160.

25. Mishra, N., Mishra, S. and Bhagwan, P. S. K. (1998). Vaccines for small ruminants-need and development strategies. *Livestock Int.*, 2(8): 9–11.

26. Burrows, R., Mann, J. A. and Garland, A. J. M. (1981). The pathogenesis of natural and simulated natural foot-and-mouth disease infection in cattle. *J. Comp. Pathol.*, 91(4): 599–609.

27. Salt, J. S. (1993). The carrier state in foot and mouth disease-an immunological review. *British Vet. J.*, 149(3): 207–223.

28. Radostits, O. M., Blood, D. C. and Gay, C. C. (1994). Veterinary Medicine, *In: Educational Low-Priced Scheme*, pp. 965–973, Balli´ere Tindall, London, UK, 8th edition.

29. Buxton, A. and Fraser, G. (1977). *Animal Microbiology*, vol. 2, Blackwell Scientific Publications, Oxford, UK.

30. Vosloo, W., Bastos, A. D. and Kirkbride, E. (1996). Persistent infection of African buffalo (*Syncerus caffer*) with SAT type foot-and-mouth disease viruses: rate of fixation of mutations, antigenic change and interspecies transmission. *J. Gen. Virol.*, 77(7): 1457–1467.

31. Remond, M., Kaiser, C. and Lebreton, F. (2002). Diagnosis and screening of foot-and-mouth disease. *Comp. Immunol. Microbiol. Infect. Dis.*, 25(5-6): 309–320.

32. Revenson, S. and Segura, M. (1963). Multiplication of foot-and-mouth disease virus in roller tube culture BHK-21 cells of hamster kidney. *Revenue Canada Invest.*, 18: 293–299.

33. Longjam N., Sarmah A. K., Deb R., Mathapati B. S., Tayo T. and Sailo B. (2010). Isolation of foot and mouth disease virus of indian origin (north eastern region) in BHK21 clone-13 cell line from clinical samples. *Ind. J. Comp. Microbiol. Immunol. Infect. Dis.*, 31(1 and 2): 71- 72.

34. Goel, A. C. and Rai, A. (1985). Growth curve, plaque assay and inactivation studies of FMD virus subtypes O5, O1 and O6 of Indian origin. *Ind. J. Comp. Microbiol. Immunol. Infect. Dis.*, 6(1): 16–28.

35. Barteling, S. J., Wagenaar, F. and Gielkens, A. L. J. (1982). The positively charged structural virus protein (VP1) of footand- mouth disease virus (type O1) contains a highly basic part which may be involved in early virus-cell interaction. *J. Gen. Virol.*, 62(2): 357–361.

36. Darbyshire, J. H., Hedger, R. S. and Arrowsmith, E. M. (1972). Comparative complement-fixation studies with subtype strains of foot-and-mouth disease virus. *J. Hyg.*, 70(1): 171–180.

37. Rweyemamu, M. M. (1982). Developments in the biochemical and immunoassays assessment of foot-and-mouth antigen. *In:* Proceedings of the Internationals Conference on the Impact of Viral Disease on the Development of Latin American Countries and Caribbean Region, pp. 78–79, Rio de Janeiro, Brazil.

38. Rweyemamu, M. M. (1984). Antigenic variation in foot-and-mouth disease: studies based on the virus neutralization reaction. *J. Biol. Standzn.*, 12(3): 323– 337.

39. Crowther, J. R. and Abu Elzein, E. M. E. (1979). Application of the enzyme linked immunosorbent assay to the detection and identification of foot-and-mouth disease viruses. *J. Hyg.*, 83(3): 513–519.

40. Ouldridge, E. J., Barnett, P. and Rweyemamu, M. M. (1982). The relative efficiency of two ELISA techniques for the tritration of FMD antigen. *Current Topics in Vet. Med. Anim. Sci.*, 22: 142–151.

41. Hoffmann, B., Martin, B., Reid, S. M., Peter, M., Oura, C. A. L., Piet, A., van Rijn Slomka, M. J., Jill Bank Ian, H., Brown, D. J., Alexander Donald, P. and King, A. M. (2009). A review of RT-PCR technologies used in veterinary virology and disease control: Sensitive and specific diagnosis of five livestock diseases notifiable to the World Organization for Animal Health. *Vet. Microbiol.*, 139: 1-23.

42. Pattnaik, B. and Venkataramanan, R. (1989). A sandwich enzyme linked immunosorbent assay for subtype analysis of foot-and-mouth disease virus isolate. *Ind. J. Anim. Sci.*, 59: 1363–1368.

43. Lunt, R. A., Linchongsubongkoch, W. and Gleeson, L. J. (1994). A modified liquid phase (LP) blocking ELISA used to assess type O foot-and-mouth disease virus antigenic variation in Thailand. *Vet. Microbiol.*, 42(1): 79–90.

44. Moonen, P., Boonstra, J., Hakze-van der Honing, R., Boonstra-Leendertse, C., Jacobs, L. and Dekker, A. (2003). Validation of a LightCycler-based reverse transcription polymerase chain reaction for the detection of foot-and-mouth disease virus. *J. Virol. Met.*, 113(1): 35– 41.

45. Moss, A. and Haas, B. (1999). Comparison of the plaque test and reverse transcription nested PCR for the detection of FMDV in nasal swabs and probang samples. *J. Virol. Met.*, 80(1): 59–67.

46. Tam, S., Clavijo, A., Engelhard, E. K. and Thurmond, M. C. (2009). Fluorescence-based multiplex real-time RT-PCR arrays for the detection and serotype determination of foot-and-mouth disease virus. *J. Virol. Met.*, 161(2): 183–191.

47. Lomakina, N. F., Fallacara, F. and Pacciarini, M. (2004). Application of universal primers for identification of Foot-and-mouth disease virus and Swine vesicular disease virus by PCR and PCR-ELISA. *Arch. Virol.*, 149(6): 1155–1170.

48. Giridharan, P., Hemadri, D., Tosh, C., Sanyal, A. and Bandyopadhyay, S. K. (2005). Development and evaluation of a multiplex PCR for differentiation of foot-and-mouth disease virus strains native to India. *J. Virol. Met.*, 126(1-2): 1–11.

49. Longjam, N., Sarmah, A. K., Deb, R., Saxena, V. K. and Tayo, T. (2012). Comparative evaluation of three diagnostic tests for detection of foot and mouth disease virus of Indian origin. *Ind. J. Anim. Sci.*, 82(3): 233-236.

50. Mackay, I. M., Arden, K. E. and Nitsche, A. (2002). Real-time PCR in virology. *Nucleic Acids Res.*, 30(6): 1292–1305.

51. Callahan, J. D., Brown, F. and Osorio, F. A. (2002). Use of a portable real-time reverse transcriptase-polymerase chain reaction assay for rapid detection of foot-and-mouth disease virus. *J. Am. Vet. Med. Assoc.*, 220(11): 1636–1642.

52. Kessler, H. H., M¨uhlbauer, G. and Rinner, B. (2000). Detection of herpes simplex virus DNA by real-time PCR. *J. Clin. Microbiol.*, 38(7): 2638–2642.

53. Suryanarayana, V. V. S., Viswanathan, S. and Ratish, G. (1999). *E. coli* expressed proteins as diagnostic reagents for typing of foot-and-mouth disease virus. *Arch. Virol.*, 144(9): 1701–1712.

54. Lu, Z., Cao, Y. and Guo, J. (2007). Development and validation of a 3ABC indirect ELISA for differentiation of foot-and-mouth disease virus infected from vaccinated animals. *Vet. Microbiol.*, 125(1-2): 157–169.

55. Renji, R., Balamurugan, V., Saha, S. N., Reddy, G. R. and Suryanarayana, V. V. S. (2003). Expression of capsid precursor polypeptide (P1) of foot and mouth disease virus vaccine strains in pichia pastoris. *Ind. J. Biotech.*, 2(4): 533–538.

56. Ko, Y. J., Jeoung, H. Y. and Lee, H. S. (2009). A recombinant protein-based ELISA for detecting antibodies to foot-andmouth disease virus serotype Asia 1. *J. Virol. Met.*, 159(1): 112–118.

57. Uttenthal, A., Parida, S., Rasmussen, T. B., Paton, D. J., Haas, B. and Dundon, W. G. (2010). Strategies for differentiating infection in vaccinated animals (DIVA) for foot-andmouth disease, classical swine fever and avian influenza. *Expert Rev. Vaccines*, 9(1): 73–87.

58. Henderson, L. M. (2005). Overview of marker vaccine and differential diagnostic test technology. *Biologicals.*, 33(4): 203–209.

59. Fowler, V. L., Knowles, N. J., Paton, D. J. and Barnett, P. V. (2010). Marker vaccine potential of a foot-and-mouth disease virus with a partial VP1 G-H loop deletion. *Vaccine.*, 28(19): 3428–3434.

60. Baxi, M. K., Baxi, S., Clavijo, A., Burton, K. M. and Deregt, D. (2006). Microarray-based detection and typing of foot-and-mouth disease virus. *Vet. J.*, 172(3): 473–481.

61. McFarlane, R. G., Molitor, T. W. and Vakharia, V. N. (1990). The detection and differentiation of foot-and-mouth disease viruses using solid-phase nucleic acid hybridization. *J. Virol. Met.*, 27(2): 175–188.

62. Lau, L. T., Reid, S. M. and King, D. P. (2008). Detection of foot-and-mouth disease virus by nucleic acid sequence-based amplification (NASBA). *Vet. Microbiol.*, 126(1–3): 101–110.

63. Kim, Y. J., Lebreton, F., Kaiser, C., Cruci'ere, C. and R´emond, M. (2004). Isolation of foot-and-mouth disease virus specific bovine antibody fragments from phage display libraries. *J. Immunol. Met.*, 286(1-2): 155–166.

64. Reid, S. M., Ferris, N. P., Br¨uning, A., Hutchings, G. H., Kowalska, Z. and Akerbolm, L. (2001). Development of a rapid chromatographic strip test for the pen-side detection of foot-and-mouth disease virus antigen. *J. Virol. Met.*, 96(2): 189–202.

65. Dukes, J. P., King, D. P. and Alexandersen, S. (2006). Novel reverse transcription loop-mediated isothermal amplification for rapid detection of foot-and-mouth disease virus. *Arch. Virol.*, 151(6): 1093–1106.

66. Aarthi, D., Rao, K. A., Robinson, R. and Srinivasan, V. A. (2004). Validation of binary ethelyneimine (BEI) used as an inactivant for foot and mouth disease tissue culture vaccine. *Biological.*, 32: 153-156.

67. Srinivasan, V. A. FMD vaccines and vaccination in India; Production, use and quality. Indian Immunologicals Limited, Hyderabad- 500 032.

68. Venkataraman, R. India: Foot and mouth disease control initiatives. I.V.R.I, Bangalore.

69. Kiran, K. K, Ravi, P. and Prabhudas, K. (2005). Infectious bovine rhnotracheitis- National survey of IBR antibodies by AB-ELISA kit. Annual Report of Project Directorate on Animal Disease Monitoring and Surveillance, ICAR, Bangalore 7-10.

70. Mehrotra, M. L. (1977). Isolation of respiratory viruses from cattle and their possible role in genital disorders. PhD thesis, Agra University, Agra.

71. Suribabu, T., Mallick, B. B. and Das, S. K. (1984). Prevalence of IBR virus (BHV-1) antibodies in bovines. *Ind. Vet. J.*, 61: 195-200.

72. Metzler, A. E., Matile, H., Gassmann, U., Engels, M. and Wyler, R. (1985). European isolates of bovine herpesvirus 1: a comparison of restriction endonuclease sites, polypeptides, and reactivity with monoclonal antibodies. *Arch. Virol.*, 85: 57–69.

73. Edwards, S., White, H. and Nixon, P. (1990). A study of the predominant genotypes of bovid herpesvirus 1 isolated in the U.K. *Vet. Microbiol.*, 22: 213–223.

74. Magyar, G., Tanyi, J., Hornyak, A. and Batha, A. (1993). Restriction endonuclease analysis of Hungarian bovine herpesvirus isolates from different clinical forms of IBR, IPV and encephalitis. *Acta Vet. Hung.*, 41: 159–170.

75. Thirty, J., Keuser, V., Muylkens, B., Meurens, F., Gogev, S. and Vanderplasschen, A. and Thiry, E. (2006). Ruminant alphaherpesviruses related to bovine herpesvirus 1. *Vet. Res.*, 37: 169–190.

76. Mechor, G. D., Rousseaux, C. G., Radostits, O. M., Babiuk, L.A. and Petrie, L. (1987). Protection of newborn calves against fatal multisystemic infectious bovine rhinotracheitis by feeding colostrum from vaccinated cows. *Can. J. Vet. Res.*, 51: 452–459.

77. Suresh, K. B., Sudharshana, K. J. and Rajasekar, M. (1999). Seroprevalence of infectious bovine rhinotracheitis in India. *Ind. Vet. J.*, 76(1): 5-9.

78. Van Oirschot, J. T., Straver, P. J., Van Lieshout, J. A. H., Quak, J., Westenbrink, F. and Van Exsel, A. C. A. (1993). A subclinical infection of bulls with bovine herpesvirus type 1 at an artificial insemination centre. *Vet. Rec.*, 132: 32–35.

79. Brunner, D., Engels, M., Schwyzer, M. and Wyler, R. (1988). A comparison of three techniques for detecting bovine herpesvirus type 1 (BHV-1) in naturally and experimentally contaminated bovine semen. *Zuchthygiene.*, 23: 1–9.

80. Kaashoek, M. J., Moerman, A., Madic, J., Rijsewijk, F. A. M., Quak, J., Gielkens, A. L. J. and Van Oirschot, J. T. (1994). A conventionally attenuated glycoprotein E-negative strain of bovine herpesvirus type 1 is an efficacious and safe vaccine. *Vaccine*, 12: 439–444.

81. Edwards, S., Chasey, D. and White, H. (1983). Experimental infectious bovine rhinotracheitis: comparison of four antigen detection methods. *Res. Vet. Sci.*, 34: 42–45.

82. Lemaire, M., Weynants, V., Godfroid, J., Schynts, F., Meyer, G., Letesson, J. J. and Thiry, E. (2000). Effects of bovine herpesvirus type 1 infection in calves with maternal antibodies on immune response and virus latency. *J. Clin. Microbiol.*, 38 (5): 1885–1894.

83. Office des International Epizootics. (2010). Infectious Bovine Rhinotracheitis/Infectious Pustular Vulvovaginitis. Adopted version of the World assembly of delegates of the OIE. Chapter 2.4.13.

84. Wellenberg, G. J., Verstraten, E. R. A. M., Mars, M. H. and Van Oirschot, J. T. (1998a). Detection of bovine herpesvirus 1 glycoprotein E antibodies in individual milk samples by enzyme-linked immunosorbent assays. *J. Clin. Microbiol.*, 36: 409–413.

85. Frankena, K., Franken, P., Vandehoek, J., Koskamp, G. and Kr amps, J. A. (1997). Probability of detecting antibodies to bovine herpesvirus 1 in bulk milk after the introduction of a positive animal on to a negative farm. *Vet. Rec.*, 140: 90–92.

86. Wellenberg, G. J., Verstraten, E. R. A. M., Mars, M. H. and Van Oirschot, J. T. (1998b). ELISA detection of antibodies to glycoprotein E of bovine herpesvirus 1 in bulk milk samples. *Vet Rec.*, 142: 219–220.

87. Nylin, B., Stroger, U. and Ronsholt, L. (2000). A retrospective evaluation of a bovine herpesvirus-1 (BHV-1) antibody ELISA on bulk-tank milk samples for classification of the BHV-1 status of Danish dairy herds. *Prev. Vet. Med.*, 47: 91–105.

88. Babu, N. G. R. and Rajasekhar, M. (1988). Prevalence of rinderpest antibodies in sheep and goats in southern India. *Vet. Rec.*, 123 (23): 595-597.

89. Perrin, B., Bitsch, V., Cordioli, P., Edwards, S., Eloit, M., Guerin, B., Lenihan, P., Perrin, M., Ronsholt, L., Van Oirschot, J. T., Vanopdenbosch, E., Wellemans, G., Wizigmann, G. and Thibier, M. (1993). A European comparative study of serological methods for the diagnosis of infectious bovine rhinotracheitis. *Rev. sci. tech. Off. int. Epiz.*, 12: 969–984.

90. Fuchs, M., Hubert, P., Detterer, J. and Rziha, H. J. (1999). Detection of bovine herpesvirus type 1 in blood from naturally infected cattle by using a sensitive PCR that discriminates between wild-type virus and virus lacking glycoprotein E. *J. Clin. Microbiol.*, 37: 2498–2507.

91. Ros, C., Riquelme, M. E., Ohman Forslund, K. and Belak, S. (1999). Improved detection of five closely related ruminant alpha herpes viruses by specific amplification of viral genome sequences. *J. Virol. Met.*, 83: 55–65.

92. Van Engelenburg, F. A. C., Van Schie, F. W., Rijsewijk, F. A. M. and Van Oirschot, J. T. (1995). Excretion of bovine herpesvirus 1 in semen is detected much longer by PCR than by virus isolation. *J. Clin. Microbiol.*, 33: 308–312.

93. Grom, J., Hostnik, P., Toplak, I. and Barlic-Maganja, D. (2006). Molecular detection of BHV-1 in artificially inoculated semen and in the semen of a latently infected bull treated with dexamethasone. *Vet. J.*, 171: 539–544.

94. Mars, M. H., De Jong, M. C. M., Franken, P. and Van Oirschot, J. T. (2001). Efficacy of a live glycoprotein E-negative bovine herpesvirus 1 vaccine in cattle in the field. *Vaccine*, 19: 1924–1930.

95. Flewett, T. H. and Woode, G. N. (1978). The rotaviruses. Brief review. *Arch. Virol.*, 57: 1-23.

96. Pastoret, P. P., Schwers, A., Vanden Broecke, C. and Werenne, J. (1984). Epizootiology of rotavirus diarrhoea in the bovine specie. *Rev. sci. tech. Off. Int. Epiz.*, 3(4): 843-853.

97. Ciarlet, M. and Estes, M. K. (1999). Human and most animal rota virus strains do not require the presence of sialic acid on the cell surface for efficient infectivity. *J. Gen. Virol.*, 80: 943-948.

98. Kapikian, A. Z., Hoshino, Y. and Chanock, R. M. (2001). Rotaviruses. *Fields Virol.*, 4th Edn. Lippincott Williams and Wilkins, London, pp. 1787-1833.

99. Desselberger, U. (1998). Reoviruses. *In:* Collier L, Balow A, Sussman M, editors. *Topley and Wilson's microbiology and microbial infections,* 9th edn, vol 1. London: Arnold; pp. 537-550.

100. Estes, M. K. (2001). Rotaviruses and their replication. *In:. Fields Virol.*, (Knipe, D. M. and Howley, P. M., eds). Lippincott-Roven Publishers, Philadelphia, 1747-1785.

101. Estes, M. K. and Cohen, J. (1989). Rotavirus gene structure and function. *Microbiol. Rev.*, 53(4): 410-449.

102. Das S., Sen A., Uma G., Varghese V., Chaudhuri S., Bhattacharya S.K., Krishnan T., Dutta P., Dutta D., Bhattacharya M.K., Mitra U., Kobayashi N. and Naik T.N. (2002). Genomic diversity of group A rotavirus strains infecting humans in eastern India. *J. Clin. Microbiol.*, 40(1): 146-149.

103. Fukai K., Maeda Y., Fujimoto K., Itou T. and Sakai T. (2002). Changes in the prevalence of rotavirus G and P types in diarrhoeic calves from the Kagoshima prefacture in Japan. *Vet. Microbiol.*, 86(4): 343-349.

104. Okada N. and Matsumoto Y. (2002). Bovine rotavirus G and P types and sequence analysis of the VP7 gene of two G8 bovine rotaviruses from Japan. *Vet. Microbiol.*, 84(4): 297-305.

105. Gulati, B. R., Nakagomi, O., Koshimura, Y., Nakagomi, T. and Pandey, R. (1999). Relative frequencies of G and P types among rotaviruses from Indian diarrhoeic cows and buffalo calves. *J. Clin. Microbiol.*, 37(6): 2074-2076.

106. Gulati, R. B., Maherchandani, S. and Pandey, R. (1995). Electropherotyping of genomic RNA of rotavirus from diarrhoeic calves. *Ind. J. Virol*, 11: 7-12.

107. http:// www.pathomicro.med.sc.edu.

108. Dagenais, L., Lansival, B., Pastoret, P. P., Massip, A. and Kaeckenbeeck, A. (1980a). Absence de rotavirus dans le meconium de veaux. *Ann. Méd. Vét.*, 124: 303.

109. Vanden Broecke, C., Schwers, A., Pastoret, P. P., Maenhoudt, M., De Boeck, A., Goossens, A. and Werenne, J. (1984a). Induction of interferon in colostrum-deprived new-born calves after experimental infection with bovine rotavirus. CEC Workshop on adjuvants, interferon and non-specific immunity, Venice, 27-28 April, 1983, Cancellotti F.M., Galassi D, Eds. Office for official publications of the European Communities, Luxembourg, 45.

110. Dagenais, L., Pastoret, P. P., Massip, A., Kaeckenbeeck, A. and Lansival, B. (1981). Failure to isolate rotavirus from bovine meconium. *Vet. Rec.*, 108: 11.

111. Schlaffer, D. H., Schultz, R. D., Scott, F. W. and Duncan, J. R. (1979). Bovine fetal inoculations with calf rotavirus. *Can. J. Comp. Med.*, 43: 405.

112. Mc Nulty, M. S., Mc Ferran, J. B., Bryson, D. G., Logan, F. F. and Curran, W. L. (1976). Studies on rotavirus infection and diarrhea in young calves. *Vet. Rec.*, 99: 229.

113. Dagenais, L., Pastoret, P. P., Schwers, A., Kaeckenbeeck, A., Lansival, B., Antoine, H., Joassin, L., Calberg-Bacq, C. M. and Jacquemin, E. (1980b). Epizootiologie de la diarrhée à rotavirus chez les bovins. *Ann. Méd. Vét.*, 124: 565.

114. Van Opdenbosch, E., Wellemans, G., Dekegel, D. and Strobbe, R. (1979). Neonatal calf diarrhoea: a complex viral etiology. *V1. Diergeneesk. Tijdschr.*, 48: 512.

115. Scherrer, R., Cohen, J., L'Haridon, R., Feynerol, C. and Fayet, J. C. (1976). Reovirus-like agent (rotavirus) associated with neonatal calf gastroenteritis in France. *Ann. Rech. Vét.*, 7: 25.

116. Schwers, A., Mahin, L., Pastoret, P. P., Dewulf, M., Mazouz, A., Maenhoudt, M. and Michaux, C. (1984). Prevalence of antibody to rotavirus in Moroccan cattle. *Comp. Immunol. Microbiol, infect. Dis.*, 7: 69.

117. Woode, G. N. (1978). Epizootiology of bovine rotavirus infection. *Vet. Rec*, 103: 44.

118. Hoyois, P., Schwers, A. and Pastoret, P. P. (1982). Isolement de rotavirus de matières fécales de chiens de ferme maintenus en contact avec des bovins. *Ann. Méd. Vét.*, 126: 335.

119. Schwers, A., Pastoret, P. P., Dagenais, L., Maenhoudt, M., Chappuis, G., Hoyois, P., Vanden Broecke, C., Werenne, J., Massip, A., Lansival, B. and Antoine, H. (1983). Epidémiologie de la diarrhée à rotavirus dans l'espèce bovine. *Ann. Méd. Vét.*, 127: 81.

120. Vanden Broecke, C., Schwers, A., Dagenais, L., Goossens, A., Maenhoudt, M., Pastoret, P. P. and Werenne, J. (1984b). — Interferon response in colostrumdeprived newborn calves infected with bovine rotavirus: its possible role in the control of the pathogenicity. *Ann. Rech. Vet.*, 15: 29.

121. Snodgrass, D. R., Herring, J. A. and Gray, E. W. (1976). Expérimental rotavirus infection of lambs. *J. Comp. Pathol.*, 86: 637.

122. Bridger, J. C. (1980). Rotavirus: the present situation in farm animals. *Vet. Annu.*, 20: 172.

123. Tzipori, S., Makin, T. J., Smith, M. L. and Krautil, F. L. (1981). Clinical manifestations of diarrhea in calves infected with rotavirus and enterotoxigenic *Escherichia coli. J. Clin. Microbiol.*, 13: 1011.

124. Kapikian, A. Z., Kim, H. W., Wyatt, R. G., Cline, W. L, Arrobio, J. O. and Brandt, C. D. (1976). Human reovirus like-agent as the major pathogen associated with "winter" gastroenteritis in hospitalized infants and young children. *N Engl J Med.*, 294: 965-72.

125. Singh, V., Broor, S. and Mehta, S. (1986). Comparison of reverse passive haemagglutination assay and solid phase agglutination of coated erythrocytes with ELISA for rotavirus antigen detection. *Ind. J. Med. Res.*, 1986: 84: 327-330.

126. Dar, V. S., Ghosh, S. and Broor, S. (1994). Rapid detection of rotavirus by using colloidal gold particles labeled with monoclonal antibody. *J. Virol. Met.*, 47: 51-58.

127. Cukor, G. and Blacklow, N. R. (1984). Human viral gastroenteritis. *Microbiol. Rev.*, 48: 157-179.

128. Coulson, B. S., Gentsch, J. R., Das, B. K., Bhan, M. K. and Glass, R. I. (1999). Comparison of enzyme immunoassay and reverse transcriptase PCR for identification of serotype G9 rotaviruses. *J. Clin. Microbiol.*, 37: 3187-3193.

129. Jindal, S. R., Maiti, N. K. and Oberoi, M. S. (2000). Genomic diversity and prevalence of *Rotavirus* in cow and buffalo calves in northern India. *Rev. sci. tech. Off. Int. Epiz.*, 19(3): 871-876.

130. Dash, S. K., Tewari, A., Kumar, K., Goel, A. and Bhatia, A. K. (2011). Detection of rota virus from diarrhoeic cow calves in Mathura, India. *Vet. World.*, 4(12): 554-556.

131. Herring, A. J., Inglis, N. F., Ojeh, C. K., Snodgrass, D. R. and Menzies, J. D. (1981). Rapid diagnosis of rotavirus infection by direct detection of human and bovine rotavirus in stools: Comparison with electron microscopy, immunoelectroosmophoresis and fluorescent antibody technique. *J. Med. Virol.*, 7: 29-40.

132. Husain, M., Seth, P. and Broor, S. (1995). Detection of group A rotavirus by reverse transcriptase and polymerase chain reaction in feces from children with acute gastroenteritis. *Arch. Virol.*, 140: 1225-1233.

133. Snodgrass, D. R. and Wells, P. W. (1978). Passive immunity in rotaviral infections. *J.A.V.M.A.*, 173: 565.

134. Mc Nulty, M. S. (1978). Rotaviruses. J. *Gen. Virol.*, 40: 1.

135. La Bonnardiere, C., Cohen, J. and Contrepois, M. (1981). Interferon activity on rotavirus infected newborn calves. Ann. *Rech. Vét.*, 12: 8.

136. Werenne, J. (1982). L'interféron: perspectives actuelles. *Ann. Méd. Vét.*, 12(6): 93.

137. Flewett, T. H. and Woode, G. N. (1978). The rotaviruses: brief review. *Arch. Virol.*, 57: 1.

138. Snodgrass, D. R., Ojeh, C. K., Campbell, I. and Herring, A. J. (1984). Bovine rotavirus serotypes and their significance for immunization. *J. Clin. Microbiol.*, 20(3): 342-346.

139. Van Opdenbosch, E., Wellemans, G. and Broes, A. (1982). Prévention des diarrhées néonatales du veau: traitement de jeunes veaux avec du lait de vaches vaccines au moyen d'un vaccin anti-rotavirus inactivé adjuvé. *Ann. Méd. Vét.*, 126: 157-162.

140. Josse, M., Schoenaers, F. and Kaeckenbeeck, A. (1979). Inhibition de l'action de l'entérotoxine thermostable (ST) *Escherichia coli* par le sou-salicylate de bismuth. *Ann. Méd. Vét.*, 123: 481.

141. Blanton, J. D., Palmer, D., Christian, K. A. and Rupprecht, C. E. (2010). Rabies surveillance in the United States during 2009. *J. Am. Vet. Med. Assn.*, 237(6): 646-657.

142. Badrane, H., Bahloul, C., Perrin, P. and Tordo, N. (2001). Evidence of two Lyssavirus phylogroups with distinct pathogenicity and immunogenicity. *J. Virol.*, 75: 3268–3276.

143. http://www.microbeworld.org

144. Catherine, M. B. (2011). *Compendium of animal rabies prevention and control.* National Association of State Public Health Veerinarians, Inc.

145. Bradford, S. (1996). Large Animal Internal Medicine. Second Edn. Mosby. pp. 1024-1028.

146. Barrat, J. and Blancou, J. (1988). Technique simplifiée de prélèvement, de conditionnement et d'expédition de matière cérébrale pour le diagnostic de rage. *Doc. WHO/Rab. Res.*/88.27.

147. Montano Hirose, J. A., Bourhy, H. and Sureau, P. (1991). Retro-orbital route for brain specimen collection for rabies diagnosis. *Vet. Rec.*, 129: 291–292.

148. Lembo, T., Niezgoda, M., Velasco-Villa, A., Cleaveland, S., Ernest, E. and Rupprecht, C. E. (2006). Evaluation of a direct, rapid immunohistochemical test for rabies diagnosis. *Emerg. Infect. Dis.*, 12(2): 310–313.

149. Xu, G., Weber, P., Hu, Q., Xue, H., Audry, L., Li, C., Wu, J. and Bourhy, H. (2007). A simple sandwich ELISA (WELYSSA) for the detection of lyssavirus nucleocapsid in rabies suspected specimens using mouse monoclonal antibodies. *Biologicals.*, 35: 297–302.

150. Kang, B., Oh, J., Lee, C., Park, B. K., Park, Y., Hong, K., Lee, K., Cho, B. and Song, D. (2007). Evaluation of a rapid immunodiagnostic test kit for rabies virus. *J. Virol. Met.*, 145: 30–36.

151. Rudd, R. J. and Trimachi, C. V. (1989). Development and evaluation of an *in vitro* virus isolation procedure as a replacement for the mouse inoculation test in rabies diagnosis. *J. Clin. Microbiol.*, 27: 2522–2528.

152. Fooks, A. R., Johnson, N., Freuling, C. M., Wakeley, P. R., Banyard, A. C., Mc Elhinney, L. M., Marston, D. A., Dastjerdi, A., Wright, E., Weiss, R. A. and Muller, T. (2009). Emerging technologies for the detection of rabies virus: challenges and hopes in the 21st century. *PLoS Negl. Trop. Dis.*, 3: e530.

153. World Health Organization Expert Committee on Rabies, 8th Report (2005). World Health Organisation, WHO Technical Report Series, 931: WHO, Geneva, Switzerland, pp. 1–87.

154. Hooper, D. C., Morimoto, K., Bette, M., Weihe, E., Koprowski, H. and Dietzschold, B. (1998). Collaboration of antibody and inflammation in clearance of rabies virus from the central nervous system. *J. Virol.*, 72: 3711–3719.

155. Servat, A., Feyssaguet, M., Blanchard, I., Morize, J. L., Schereffer, J. L., Boue, F. and Cliquet, F. (2007). A quantitative indirect ELISA to monitor the effectiveness of rabies vaccination in domestic and wild carnivores. *J. Immunol. Met.*, 318: 1–10.

156. Council of State and Territorial Epidemiologists. Public Health Reporting and National Notification for Animal Rabies. Infectious Disease Positions Statements (2009). CSTE, Atlanta, GA. http://www.cste.org/ps2009/09-ID-12.pdf.

157. Blanton, J. D., Palmer, D., Christian, K. A. and Rupprecht, C. E. (2009). Rabies surveillance in the United States during 2009. *J. Am. Vet. Med. Assn.*, 237(6): 646-657.

158. National Animal Control Association guidelines. http://www.nacanet. org/ guidelines.html.

159. Wertheim, H. F. L., Nguyen, T. Q. and Nguyen, K. A. T. (2009). Furious rabies after an atypical exposure. *PLoS Med.*, 6(3): 264-268.

160. Ante-mortem inspection. In: U.S. Meat and Poultry Inspection Program. (1973). Meat and poultry inspection manual. Washington, D.C.: U.S. Government Printing Office; pp. 314.

161. Brochier, B., Kieny, M. P., Costy, F., Coppens, P., Bauduin, B., Lecocq, J. P., Langiet, B., Chappuis, G., Desmettre, P., Afiademanyo, K., Libois, R. and Pastoret, P. P. (1991). Large-scale eradication of rabies using recombinant vacciniarabies vaccine. *Nature.*, 354: 520–522.

162. Prasad, G., Jain, N. C. and Gupta, Y. (1992). Blue tongue virus infection in India: A review. *Rev. sci. tech. Off. Int. Epiz.*, 11(3): 699-711.

163. Roy, P., Marshall, J. J. A. and French, T. J. (1990). Structure of Bluetongue virus genome and its encoded proteins. *In:* Roy, P., Gorman, B.M. (Eds.), Current Topics in Microbiology and Immunology. Springer, Berlin.

164. Roy P. (1992). Bluetongue virus proteins. *J. Gen. Virol.*, 73: 3051–3064.

165. Han, Z. and Harty, R. N. (2004). The NS3 protein of Bluetongue virus exhibits viroporin-like properties. *J. Biol. Chem.*, 279: 43092–43097.

166. Bonneau, K. R., Zhang, N., Zhu, J., Zhang, K., Xiao, L., Xiang, W. and Mc Lachlan, N.J. (1999). Sequence comparison of the L2 and S10 genes of Bluetongue viruses from the United States and the People's Republic of China. *Virus Res.*, 61: 153–160.

167. Bonneau, K. R., Mullens, B. A. and Mc Lachlan, N. J. (2001). Occurrence of genetic drift and founder effect during quasispecies evolution of the VP2 and NS3/NS3A genes of Bluetongue virus upon passage between sheep, cattle, and *Culicoides sonorensis*. *J. Virol.*, 75: 8298–8305.

168. Anon. (1978). Annual report of the Indian Veterinary Research Institute. IVRI, Mukteswar, pp. 120.

169. Sharma, M. M., Lonkar, P. S., Srivastava, C. P., Dubey, S. C., Maru, A. and Kalra, D. B. (1985). Epidemiology of bluetongue in sheep at an organised farm in semi arid part of Rajasthan. *Ind. J. Comp. Microbiol. Immunol, Infect. Dis.*, 6:188-192.

170. Mehrotra, M. L. and Shukla, D. C. (1984). Seroprevalence of bluetongue virus in sheep, cattle and buffaloes in India. *Ind. J. Anim. Sci.*, 54: 718-719.

171. Gupta, Y., Chand, P., Shingh, A. and Jain, N. C. (1990). Dot immuno-binding assay in comparison with enzyme linked immunosorbent assay for detection of bluetongue virus antibodies in sheep. *Vet. Microbiol.*, 22: 365 371.

172. Mahajan, N. K., Prasad, G., Jain, N. C., Dhanda, J. S. and Gupta, Y. (1991). Epizootiological studies on bluetongue at an organised sheep breeding farm near Hisar, Haryana. *Ind. J. Anim. Sci.*, 61: 15.

173. Mc Phee, D. A., Parsonson, I. M. and Della Porta, A. J. (1982). Comparative studies on the growth of Australian bluetongue virus serotypes in continuous cell lines and embryonated chicken eggs. *Vet. Microbiol.*, 7: 401-410.

174. Pearson, J. E. and Jochim, M. M. (1979). Protocol for the immunodiffusion test for bluetongue. *Proc. Ann. Meet. Am. Ass. vet. lab. Diagnost.*, 22: 463-471.

175. Chander, S., Prasad, G. and Jain, N. C. (1991). Dot-immuno-binding assay for the detection of bluetongue virus antibodies in sheep experimentally inoculated with bluetongue virus serotype 1. *Vet. Microbiol.*, 28: 289-294.

176. Orru, G., Ferrando, M. L., Meloni, M., Liciardi, M., Savini, G. and Santis, P. D. (2006). Rapid detection and quantitation of Blue tongue virus (BTV) using a Molecular Beacon fluorescent probe assay. *J. Virol. Met.*, 137: 34-42.

177. Tyagi, S., Bratu, D. P. and Kramer, F. R. (1998). Multicolor Molecular Beacons for allele discrimination. *Nat. Biotechnol.*, 16: 49–53.

178. Bhanuprakash, V., Indrani, B. K., Hosamani, M., Balamurugan, V. and Singh, R. K. (2009). Blue tongue vaccines: the past, present and future. *Expert Rev. Vaccines.*, 8(2): 191-204.

□□□

Chapter 5

Major Parasitic Diseases of Cattle

5.1. Trypanosomiasis/Surra

5.1.1. Introduction

Trypanosomiasis/Surra caused by *Trypanosoma evansi* is the most widely distributed pathogenic mechanically transmitted vector borne haemoprotozoan disease of cattle in India under list B of the Office International Epizooties. Surra is responsible for causing severe anaemia, oedema, immunosuppression and various neurological disorders resulting into death of the affected animals. It is a potential killer disease of cattle in India. The disease has a major economic impact in India, but it is difficult to assess the economic losses because of non-availability of the exact epidemiological data. It is likely that the number of cases reported to the government reflect only outbreaks where mortality is high. Actual figures may be much higher than those reported due to misdiagnosis, poor monitoring and subsequently faulty reporting. Actual cases and death caused by surra may be more than five times than those reported. Most of the direct losses in the animals are there due to mortality and cost of chemotherapeutic interventions. The indirect losses due to infection have not been adequately defined, but remained an important factor in the field due to failure of vaccination against bacterial and viral infections, due to severe immunosuppression produced by the disease (Holmes 1980). Further losses are occurring through reduced yield of milk, reduced weight-gain in animals grown for meat and reduced ability shown by the draught animals.

5.1.2. Etiological agent

T. evansi is a member of subgenus *Trypanozoon* and is described as monomorphic but may be pleomorphic in some strains with length of 15 to 34 ìm. Leaf-like slender forms are characterized by a long free flagellum with narrow and drawn out posterior end. Kinetoplast is terminal or subterminal in position. Dyskinetoplastic forms also appear after treatment of *T. evansi* with a variety of trypanocidal drugs including berenil.

5.1.3. Epidemiology and transmission

The disease is endemic throughout India particularly in low-lying areas. The yearly epidemiological distribution is unsystematically reported. Cases are encountered throughout the year but the incidence is higher during rainy and post rainy seasons due to predominance of *Tabanus* flies. The incidence of surra is higher in north and northwestern parts as compared to eastern and southern parts of India. India is thought to be the major source from where surra has spread within livestock throughout the continent of Asia and Islands of Indian Ocean. Since biting flies mainly transmits *T. evansi* and infected animals are reservoirs, the disease is responsible for inhibiting the livestock movement and trade of animals. Clinical infection is frequently encountered in cows. (Aulakh 2003).

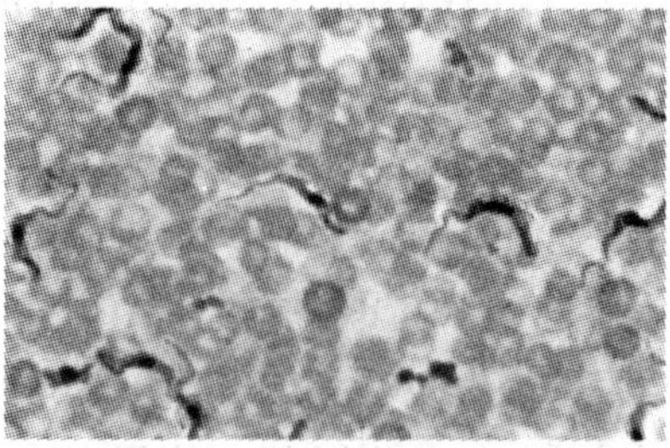

Fig. 21 : Leaf like slender form of *T. evansi* with terminal and subterminal kinetoplast (http://www.tolweb.org)

It is generally known that *T. evansi* is transmitted by various species of *Tabanus* flies. No development takes place inside the vector. Efficiency of transmission is dependent on the interval between 2 successive feedings and intensity of fly challenge. The transmission with tabanid flies is achieved mostly by interrupting feeding habit leading to transfer of infection to healthy animals. This mode has been termed as direct transmission. Tabanids are pool feeders. They cut the skin with their mouthparts and lap pooled blood along with connective tissue fluid. As a result the parasitaemia in jugular blood may not be a good indicator of infectivity for *Tabanus* transmission. Rather, the trypanosome density in capillary blood, lymph or connective tissue in the skin are more important. After feeding on infective animal when the flies take rest, the transmissions in healthy animals are successful in some cases. Surra is also known as 'makhi ki bimari' (horse fly disease) in northern states of India like Punjab and occurrs in the habitat most favourable to tabanidae. The outbreaks are most common when the flies are most numerous. For infection trypanosomes must survive in the gut of tabanids and be regurgitated during subsequent feeding. Increase in tabanid activity is expected to increase the likelihood of *T. evansi* transmission and hence contribute towards disease outbreaks during rainy and post rainy seasons.

Other blood-sucking insects, which can transmit the infections, include *Stomoxys, Lyperosia, Hematopota* (flies) and *Ornithodorus* (tick). There is some controversy concerning the ability of *Stomoxys calcitrans* to transmit *T. evansi*. *Stomoxys niger* and *Stomoxys taeniatus* are capable of transmitting *T. evansi* under laboratory conditions (Sumba *et al.*, 1998). An attempt had been made previously to transmit the disease through *Hyalomma anatolicum anatolicum* ticks in rabbit but no parasitaemia was observed (Sridhar and Sharma 1989). Another probable route of transmission is iatrogenic transmission. As the mouthparts of tabanid flies can trap only 10 nl of fluid/blood, so iatrogenic transmission such as during herd vaccination can be an important mode of spread of disease.

5.1.4. Pathogenesis

T. evansi is a blood protozoa but visceral forms have also been reported in heart, optic lobes, cerebrum, liver, kidney and lungs. Course of infection and degree of pathogencity depends upon the virulence of *T. evansi* strain. During *T. evansi* infection circulating or bound autoantibodies against erythrocytes have not been detected in rats. However, anaemia is attributed to immunological reactions. It is possible that erythrocytes may acquire trypanosomal antigen resulting in the immunological reaction and complement mediated destruction of erythrocytes. Experimentally human serum was found to be trypanolytic. However, this activity is transient in nature (Juyal *et al.*, 1998). Loss of sialic acid from erythrocytic membranes of *T. evansi*-infected cows may predispose the erythrocytes for phagocytosis and development of anaemia (Walia *et al.*, 1996). The lysosomal secretory proteinases, phospholipases and other hydrolytic enzymes of trypanosomes are considered potentially important factors in the development of the diseases caused by trypanosomes. The E/S proteases released into the blood stream may degrade the host tissue proteins and contribute to the pathogenesis. Besides causing disease, the trypanosomes are also responsible for producing a state of severe immunosuppression, which renders the infected host more susceptible to secondary infections and produce poor immune response to bacterial and viral vaccines (Touratier 1996). Immunosuppression has been shown in *T. evansi*-infected mice (Juyal and Tiwari 1982). Substantial immunosuppressive effect to Haemorrhagic Septicaemia (HS) vaccination has been recorded in experimental *T. evansi* infection in calves (Singla *et al.*, 2001).

5.1.5. Clinical signs and post mortem lesions

The clinical signs include high fever, dyspnoea, paraplegia, emaciation, keratitis, conjunctivitis, improper gait, circling along with oedema of the dependentpart of the body. There is a decrease in packed cell volume, total platelet count, erythrocytes count and hemoglobin. There may be an increase in SGOT, SGPT and globulin in *T. evansi* infected calves (Gupta *et al.*, 2003).

At post mortem, the carcass becomes emaciated with gelatinous exudates in the subcutaneous region. Spleenomegally, congestion of abomasums and intestine along with petechiae of kidney, liver and heart are among the other findings at necropsy.

5.1.6. Diagnosis

Trypanosomosis is characterized by fluctuating parasitaemia with periods of paroxysms and intermission. Though several diagnostic techniques exist for diagnosis of surra. Only few tests have been critically evaluated and standardized and still fewer are currently used routinely in India. Conventional parasitological techniques (CPT) followed in India include wet blood film, stained thin and thick blood smears. Demonstration of trypanosomes in blood is the only true gold standard and the most commonly adopted diagnostic technique used in the laboratory. Parasites can also be found in other body fluids and tissues.

The giemsa-stained thin blood smears have a low sensitivity equivalent to 10^5 trypanosome /ml. So in case of subclinical infection, it is often difficult or impossible to demonstrate parasites in the blood mainly because of the periodically cryptic nature of the parasitaemia. More than 50 to 80 % of the infections are cryptic and undetectable by direct microscopy. Nevertheless in endemic areas where the treatment is to be administered on herd basis, even a test with low sensitivity will suffice. But it provides inadequate information on the epidemiology and magnitude of the disease in the country, making monitoring and strategic control planning difficult. So CPT cannot be relied upon for diagnosis and chemotherapy. Therefore, it is imperative to use test, which is more sensitive. The diagnostic capability can be significantly improved by adopting simple low cost alternative, the haematocrit centrifugation technique (HCT) that has sensitivity equivalent to 85 trypanosomes/ml. In some areas this test is used for detecting trypanosomes in the host blood in field conditions. Furthermore, the sensitivity of parasite detection can be enhanced ten folds by using buffy coat instead of whole blood. The miniature anion-exchange centrifugation technique is considered more sensitive method for detecting trypanosomes in the blood and is able to detect one trypanosome per two ml of the blood (Reid *et al.* 2001). Mouse inoculation (MI) test is generally regarded and accepted as the most sensitive method to detect the animal trypanosomosis. When using buffy coat for inoculating the mice, the sensitivity is further increased to one trypanosome per four ml of blood. However, the need to maintain the live animals makes this test as an impractical field tool.

Some immunological tests are used as they detect antibodies produced in response to *T. evansi* antigen. The advent of enzyme linked immunosorbent assays (ELISA) has generated greater interest in the potential of serodiagnosis in the control of surra but most of the tests used have limited success. However, these tests can be used for studying epidemiology and to monitor the effect of implementation of control strategy against trypanosomosis. Some tests like antigen based ELISA and Suratex are useful in detection of current infections (Pathak *et al.*, 1997) while antibody based ELISA and CATT (Card agglutination trypanosomal test) are useful for sero-epidemiology of cattle, buffalo and camels (Dhami *et al.*, 1999). There is a need to evaluate and validate the enzyme immunoassays for antigen or antibody for field surveys.

More recently PCR (Polymerase chain reaction) and DNA probes have been used for detection of trypanosomosis in animals and hold a ray of hope for the future (Omnawar *et al.*, 2001).

5.1.7. Prophylaxis, prevention and control

Currently available drugs in India for treatment and prophylactic use against trypanosomiasis in cattle include diminazene aceturate (Berenil 20%@8-10mg/kg body wt. i/m), Suramin (Antrypol 10%@1mg/kg body wt. i/v and quinapyramine sulphate (Triquin-S and Antrycide 20%@3-5mg/kg body wt. s/c) (Gill 1991. Diminazene diaceturate in combination with antipyrine and procaine can be employed for the treatment of trypanosomosis in cow calves @ 3.12 mg/kg body weight at 14 days intervals. This is based on the pharmacokinetic observations in experimental cow calves (Kaur 2001). Chemoprophylaxis with the above mentioned drugs should be started before the onset of rainy season, thus helping in protecting the susceptible animals during the high-risk period. Along with this, prompt treatment of the sick animals helps in reducing the risk of spread of infection and development of carrier status. Trypanocides must be selected keeping in mind the problem of drug resistance in the area.

Hopes for the development of conventional vaccines are limited due to the ability of the organism to escape the host immune response through antigenic variation. An alternate immunological approach which aims at reducing the pathological consequences of trypanosome infection through disease immunomodulation, has been used in surra. Impairment of Blood Brain Barrier (BBB) and increased intracerebral immunoglobulin biosynthesis has occurred in *T. evansi* infected cow calves and marked improvement is observed after levamisole treatment (Singla et *al.*,1998). Immunostimulatory effect of levamisole is also observed by hypergammaglobulinemia (Singla and Juyal 1992) and increased immunoglobulin production. Levamisole also produces leucocytosis and lymphocytosis in *T. evansi* infected calves to combat the disease but dexamethasone should be avoided as it flares up the disease.

The control consists of integrated approach *i.e.* proper management, chemotherapy, chemoprophylaxis and vector control. However, mass campaign for eradication of Tabanus and other biting flies by spraying insecticides has limited value under Indian condition. Thus, chemotherapy and chemoprophylaxis remains the mainstay of control of Surra in India. An integrated approach of control based on early diagnosis, treatment of sick animals, identification of endemic areas and application of chemoprophylactics agents needs to be explored for control of the disease.

5.2. Theileriosis

5.2.1. Introduction

Theileriosis is a major tick borne hemoprotozoan disease of cattle, particularly of crossbred animals. It an infectious disease characrterized by enlargement of lymph node, pulmonary oedema, haemorrhages on kidney and liver, ulcers in abomasums and cattharal enteritis. Theileriosis in Indian bovines is mainly caused by *Theileria annulata* and the disease is known as Bovine Tropical Theileriosis. The chief vector responsible for transmission is mainly *Hyalomma anatolicum anatolicum* and other ticks species belonging to this genus. Bovine Tropical Theileriosis is a serious constraint in the upgradation program (Balasubramaniam 2004) as the high yielding cattle and their crossbreds are highly susceptible to the disease.

5.2.2. Etiological agent

The genus Theileria belongs to the phylum Apicomplexa, class Sporozoasida, order Eucoccidiorida, suborder Piroplasmorina and family Babesiidae (Allsopp *et al.*, 1994). *T. annulata* sporozoite stage remains dormant in the erythrocytes in the blood circulation whereas the actively multiplying stage is the schizont that are found in the lymphocytes.

5.2.3. Epidemiology and transmission

Theileriosis is a four component system in which host, environment, parasite and vector play their role in the spread of disease (Callow *et al.*, 1976). The occurrence of tropical theileriosis is seasonal and coincides with the incidence of ticks on the host, which is very high in summer *i.e.*, from May to October. The stress due to extreme of hot climate, transportation, intercurrent disease, vaccination *etc.* are the contributory factors for the occurrence of the diseases (Brown 1997). The vector of *T. annulata, Hyalomma anatolicum anatolicum* is mainly found in desert, semi desert and steppe. It occurs from North West Africa east ward to India. It is a three host tick and both immature and adult stages occur on cattle. The adults are active in late spring. The immature stage of *H. anatolicum* feed on most of the animals and larvae and nymphs infect after molting when they feed as nymphs or adults. The transmission of theilerial particles from one stadia to another stadia takes place by a process known as transtadial transmission. The theilerial particles can not survive for longer period in the tick and hence no transovarian transmission occurs. The season of adult feeding and thus of disease incidence in widely spread from March to November, but the nymphs have a more restricted season from July to September. The seasonal incidence of *T. annulata* is commonly in late spring and early summer.

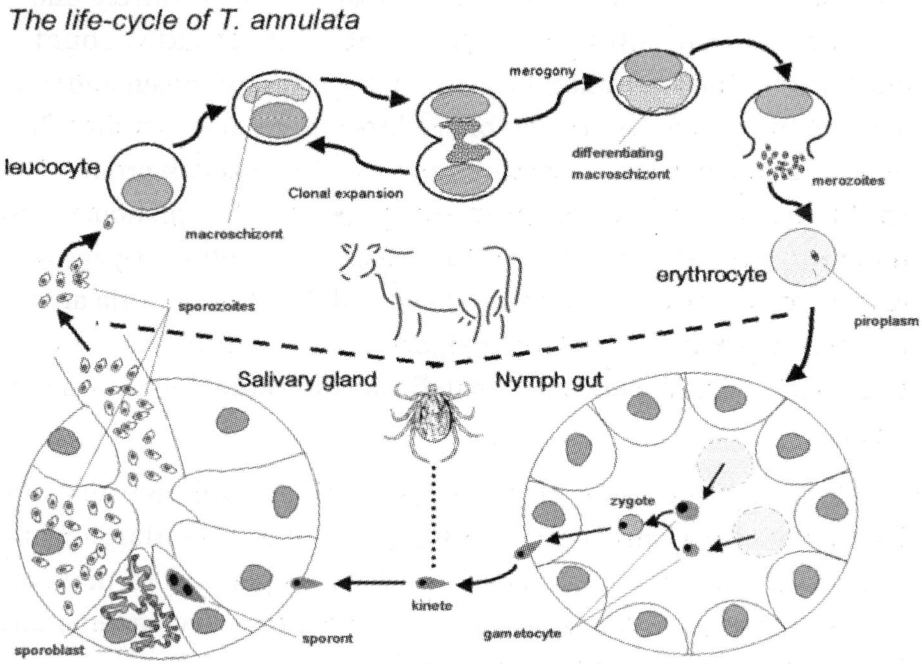

Fig. 22 : Life cycle of *T. annulata* (http://www.theileria.org.gif)

5.2.4. Pathogenesis correlating with clinical signs and post mortem lesions

Due to schizogony in the lymphoid tissue hyperplasia occurs causing swelling oflymphnodes. Due to sudden release of toxins of macroschizonts high rise in body temperature and formation of the ulcers on the mucosal layers of abomasum. In acute cases there is disponea and death due to anaemic anaemia. The disease runs peracute, acute, sub acute or chronic course. In exotic cattle, the peracute form of the disease may be noticed when the animal feeds and ruminates normally a day earlier and dies on the next day with a high rise of temperature. Death rate ranging from 10 to 90 per cent may occur. Cases of cerebral involvement may be seen.

The disease may commence with 40 to 41.7°C temperature which continues till the death or cure of the animal. The superficial lymph nodes are swollen (Bamett 1977). Leucopenia is not characteristic of the disease. There isprogressive leucocytosis which is entirely due to lymphocytes'. The RBC infection is high. The low RBC count is attributed to the removal of infected erythrocytes by spleen and liver and not due to the destruction of erythrocytes by the parasite. High fever after the tick bite, capricious appetite, drop in milk production, cessation of rumination, enlargement of superficial lymph nodes upto the size of a coconut, rough hair coat, excessive salivation, dry muzzle, respiratory distress, pulmonary oedema and haemoglobinuria are the noteable clinical signs. Nervous signs may be seen in the terminal stage of the peracute form. Ultimately, death occurs due to anaemic anoxia.

At necropsy, there may be generalized oedematous and haemorrhagic lymph nodes, the spleen may be enlarged and haemorrhagic, hepatomegally with mottled appearance of the liver, ulcers on mucosa of abomasums, massive pulmonary oedema and hyperaemia along with hydropericardium.

5.2.5. Diagnosis

Direct wet mount preparation using hypotonised erythrocytes can be employed for demonstration of the intra erythocytic forms. The demonstration of the Koch's blue bodies in the lymphocytes and monocytes of the lymph node smear or peripheral blood film by Wright's staining is pathognomonic of the disease (Jithendran 2000). Complement Fixation test, florescent antibody technique, formol gel precipitation and ELISA are among the prominent serological tests that can be employed according to the feasibility. PCR based detection of the parasite from tick collected from cattle can also aid to diagnosis (Das and Ray 2003).

5.2.6. Chemotherapy, prevention and control

Oxyteracycline@15-20mg/kg body wt. or single injection of buparvaquone@ 2.5mg.kg body wt. i/m have been used with great success in treating *Theileria* infected cattle besides the commercially available schizont vaccine Rakshavac T (to be given at 2 months of age) for prophylactic use. However, except the organised farms, use of vaccine is not popular due to higher cost and non-availability. As the transmission involves the tick vector, elimination of the vector population becomes essential for the control of theileriosis (Jithendran 1997).

5.3. Babesiosis

5.3.1. Introduction

Tick fever or cattle fever (babesiosis) is economically the most important arthropod-borne disease of cattle worldwide as well as in India. The disease is caused by intraerythrocytic protozoan parasites of the genus Babesia that infect a wide range of domestic and wild animals and occasionally man. The disease is tick transmitted and distributed worldwide. The major economic impact of babesiosis is on the cattle industry and the two most important species in cattle predominant in India are *Babesia bovis* and *B. bigemina* (Bhikane *et al.*, 2001). The main vectors of Babesia are *Boophilus* ticks which have been recently reclassified as *Rhipicephalus* species. However, it is desirable that the name *Boophilus* remains available since there is a wealth of literature on *Boophilus* species and a large part of the tick, babesia and livestock community use these names on a regular basis (Bock *et al.*, 2004). Breeds of cattle that are indigenous to Babesia endemic regions often have a certain degree of natural resistance to disease and the consequences of infection are not as serious as when exotic *Bos taurus* breeds are involved. In addition, in tropical countries like India, with a high vector population, natural exposure usually occurs at an early age and cattle are therefore immune to subsequent challenge as adults. Costs due to babesiosis are incurred not only from mortality, ill-thrift, abortions, loss of milk or meat production and draft power and from control measures such as acaricide treatments, purchase of vaccines and therapeutics, but also through its impact on international cattle trade (Mc Leod and Kristjanson 1999).

5.3.2. Etiological agent and epidemiology

The classification of *Babesia* organisms *i,e.* phylum, class, order and suborder are same as that of *Theileria* spp.

The organisms are mainly transmitted by one host tick *Boophilus microplus.* The transmission is transvorian. Once the adult female tick is infected it can transmit the infection for 32 generations 18. Hence *Babesia* are called parasites of ticks rather than of vertebrate host. Another important point is that no multiplication is known to occur in the vertebrate host. Multiplication occurs exclusively in ticks. Hence, *Babesia* can survive and propogate without the vertebrate host. Male ticks, nymph and adult female can transmit the disease.

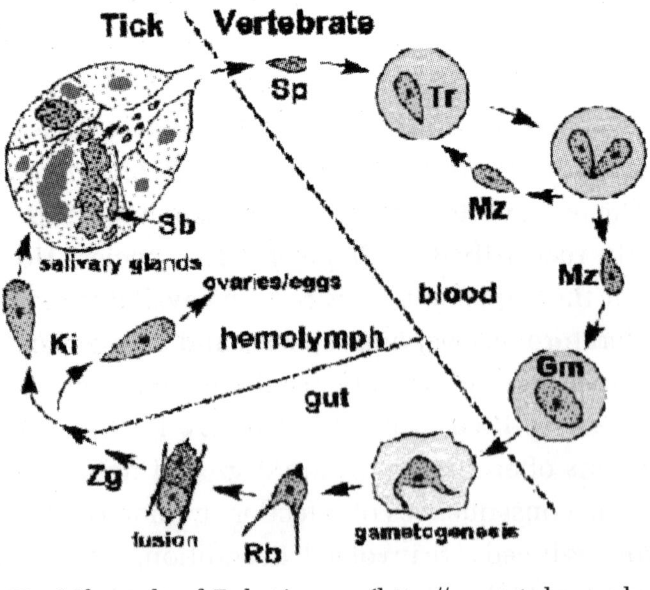

Fig. 23 : Life cycle of *Babesia* spp. (http://www.tulane.edu.gif).

The age of animal especially in the enzootic areas shows that adult animals suffer more than the young animals. Young animals have preimunition and mostly suffer from latent symptomsless infection but fetal infection in newborns are not uncommon. Sub clinical disease is more present in calves below 6 months and adults of 2 years and above (Garg *et al.,* 2004). During the summer season, when the environment is conducive for the development of ticks, the disease may raise its head. However the disease is more prevalent in monsoon season followed by summer and winter.

5.3.3. Pathogenesis

Due to infection there is anemia and icterus due to three fold loss of RBCs, heamoglobinuria due to overload of the haemoglobin in the kidneys and glomerulonephritis and heamoglobinuric nephrosis due to the immunological complexes lodged in the glomerulli and death due to organic failure. Besides the clinical manifestations, the disease can induce severe haemolytic anaemia due to heavy destruction of infected red cells, removal of non-infected erythrocytes by phagocytes, increased fragility of non infected RBC during *B. bovis* infection (Prasad 1989) and adsorption of circulating antigen antibody complexes to the surface ofRBC leading to RBC removal by phagocytosis (Sibinovic *et al.,* 1969). In addition to anaemia, detectable haematological changes include significant decrease in Hb, PCV and TEC within 48 hours of infection. Leucocytosis with neutrophilia occurs in the beginning which come dowon to normal after 12-15 days of infection. Parasitaemia is associated some what with the rise in body temperature. Substantial increase in plasma kallikrein, kinin and kininogens are due to activation of kallikrein system with an enzyme contained in *B. bovis* extracts (Mahoney 1977). Kallikrein produces vasodilation intravascular coagulation and vascular permeability, leading to circulatory stasis and shock. Increase in albumin and bile pigment has been reported during *B. bigemina* infection in cattle. Observations on blood glucose, urea nitrogen, bilirubin and transaminases indicates significant increase suggesting considerable liver damage. Central nervous system damage occurs due to concentration of parasitized cells in brain capillaries leading to obstruction of blood flow and adherence of infected cells to one another and to the vessel endothelium probably due to aparasite born antigen which alters the surface charge of RBC. There may be death of cross-bred calves manifesting symptoms like paddling of feet, grinding of teeth convulsions and coma. An important observation in such animals is distension of cerebral capillaries due to clumping of *B. bovis* parasitized erythrocytes. Haemoglobinauria and appearance of parasites in peripheral blood smears need not be necessarily present in such cases. However, when haernoglobinuria is evident *B. bovis* parasites can be detected in varying concentrations in smears from heart, kidney, liver etc. in addition to brain 25. Natural cases of cerebral babesiosis due to *B. bovis* in cross bred bovines have also been discovered (Shastri and Kulkarni 1988). The Babesiosis disease is intertransmissible from buffalo to cattle and vice versa.

5.3.4. Resistance and cross-protection to infection

Bos indicus breeds almost invariably experience milder clinical symptoms to primary *B. bovis* infections than *Bos taurus* breeds (Lohr 1973). This phenomenon is thought to be a result of the evolutionary relationship between *Bos indicus* cattle, *Boophilus* spp. and *Babesia* (Dalgliesh 1993).

Protective cross species immunity against infection cannot be induced with *B. bovis* and *B. bigemina* (Smith *et al.*, 1980). It has been noticed that *B. bovis* infection does not protect against *B. bigemina* challenge, but *B. bigemina* immunity does give some protection against *B. bovis* (Wright *et al.*, 1987).

5.3.5. Clinical signs and post mortem lesions

There is rise of temperature upto 41-45.5°C, anoxeria, increase in respiratory and heart rate, anaemia, jaundice, haemoglobinuria characterized by coffee coloured urine, either constipation or diarrhoea, weight loss abortion in pregnant animals, nervous symptoms in *Babesia bovis* infection In calves, there may be coma and death due to anaemic anoxia. Chronically affected animals may become carrier. In chronic cases, haemoglobinuria is absent.

At necropsy, there may be oedematous and yellowish subcutaneous, sub serous and intra muscular tissue, icteric discoloration of organs, enlarged liver and distended gall bladder with dark green bile. Kidneys may be enlarged and dark, lungs may be edematous, urinary bladder distended with coffee coloured urine, and characteristic intravascular cloting.

5.3.6. Diagnosis

Babesia bovis is classically known as a 'small' *Babesia* measuring up to 2 mm in diameter, while *B. bigemina* is larger and can extend to the full diameter of an erythrocyte (Potgieter 1977). Both the species show considerable morphological variation, making it difficult to identify one from the other on morphological grounds alone (De Vos and Potgieter 1994). Diagnoses of babesiosis are made by examination of blood and/or organ smears stained with Giemsa. For the best results, blood films should be prepared from capillary blood collected, for instance, after pricking the tip of the tail or margin of an ear. Labelling of parasites with fluorescein or horseradish peroxidase conjugated anti-*B. bovis* and anti- *B. bigemina* IgG is a sensitive, specific laboratory tool to identify parasites in blood and organ preparations, provided adequate numbers of parasites are present (Johnston *et al.*, 1977; Harkirat *et al.*, 2007). DNA probes are relatively sensitive tools (Bo¨se *et al.*, 1995). PCR assays, in vitro cultures and subinoculation into susceptible, usually splenectomised calves can be employed to provide a diagnosis. RAPD fingerprinting studies have also been employed for studying the DNA polymorphism of *B. bigemina* (Ravindran *et al.*, 2008). Despite the added sensitivity of these methods, stained blood or organ smears offer considerable advantages in cost and speed for clinical cases.

5.3.7. Chemotherapy, prevention and control

Currently, diminazene aceturate and imidocarb dipropionate (imidocarb) are the most widely used drugs. Diminazene works rapidly against *B. bovis* and *B. bigemina* at a dose of 3.5 mg/kg intramuscularly. It is well tolerated and will protect cattle from the two diseases for 2 and 4 weeks, respectively (De Vos 1979). Imidocarb is used subcutaneously at a dose of 1.2 mg/kg for treatment while 3 mg/kg provides protection from *B. bovis* for 4 weeks and *B. bigemina* for at least 2 months (Taylor and Mc Hardy 1979). At the high dose, imidocarb also eliminates *B. bovis* and *B. bigemina* from carrier animals.

Eradication of the tick vectors, the so-called minimum disease situation, is a permanent solution to the problem but is rarely considered practical, environmentally sustainable or economically justifiable on either a national or a local basis. Natural endemic stability can seldom be relied on as a disease control strategy. Firstly, in endemic areas, climatic effects, genetic make-up of hosts and management strategies, inevitably have a major effect on the rate of transmission and ultimately on the likelihood of endemic stability developing. Secondly, endemic stability is an economic concept that incorporates risk management and loss thresholds. The climatic, animal and management parameters that allow endemic stability can change on a seasonal, let alone on an annual, basis. For instance, a dry season can drastically affect tick numbers and parasite transmission rates to produce a generation of susceptible cattle. Livestock industries need to take a pragmatic approach to management of the ticks and diseases associated with them. In the long term, an effective outcome can be achieved by integrating the strategic use of acaricides, exploitation of endemic stability, the application of vaccines in endemically unstable conditions and the use of tick-resistant breeds of cattle (Perry *et al.*, 1998).

Both live and inactivated vaccines are available for immunizing cattle. The live vaccine is propagated in splenectomised calf by passaging around 30 times (Callow and Dalgliesh 1980). The chilled form of the attenuated vaccine is most widely used and to reduce the risk of neonatal haemolytic disease in calves of vaccinated dams, it is advised not to vaccinate cattle repeatedly and to vaccinate only young stock. RAP-1 is a 60 kDa antigen of *Babesia* that is recognised by antibodies and T cells from naturally immune cattle (Norimine *et al.*, 2002). Native and recombinant *B. bovis* and *B. bigemina* RAP-1 can confer partial protection against challenge infection.

5.4. Tick control as a measure for controlling haemoprotozoan diseases like Theileriosis and Babesiosis

Tick control is an important step in the control of bothh Theileriosis as well as Babesiosis. There are three methods of controlling the tick population *viz.*, physical, chemical and use of bio-pesticides.

5.4.1. Physical method

The physical control methods include burning of pasture at the end of grazing season, burning of cracks and crevices in the cattle shade, hunting of bushes in the grazing land, rotational grazing, zero grazing for calves and most importantly good management of calves for the first 3-6 months of life. When valuable crossbred animals are reared under confinement, a tick proof house free from cracks and crevices can be constructed. An acaricide channel should encircle the entire building and should be kept always filled with suitable acaricide solution. Fumigation of building before or at the beginning of monsoon season is essential.

5.4.2. Chemical method

Acaricides like amitraz, chlorfenvinphos, crotoxyphos, chlorphyrifos, coumaphos, cypermethrin, deltamethrin, diazinon, permethrin, phosmet, dichlorovos and trichlorophon can be used in spray, dips, slow release ear tags, leg tags and tail tags. Injection of Ivermectin at the dose rate of 200 ug *I* kg body weight s/c is effective.

At the same time, the acaricide spraying on the animal and house should be carried out.

5.4.3. Use of bio-pesticides

Combination of neem oil/extract and karanj oil at the proportion of 1:1 is effective bio-pesticide control of ticks.

5.5. Coccidiosis in calves

5.5.1. Introduction

Coccidiosis, caused by protozoa of the genus *Eimeria*, results in health and economic problems to several classes of livestock. The disease reduces feed consumption, body weight, and feed efficiency and may cause mortality of upto 25% in some cases (Fitzgerald 1975). Coccidiosis commonly affects young cattle up to 2 years of age. Animals housed in proximity are more likely to contract the disease. Therefore, feedlot and dairy cattle are most susceptible. Coccidiosis in feedlot cattle is associated with stress caused by shipping, changes in ration and in weather, and overcrowding (Ernst and Benz 1986). Stress caused by weaning makes dairy calves very susceptible to coccidiosis. It causes severe enteritis and diarrhoea. Clinical coccidiosis in cattle is normally seen in animals over 4 weeks of age.

5.5.2. Etiological agent

All domestic animal species are susceptible to coccidial infections. Although coccidia are hostspecific, each host may be infected with several species of coccidia at the same time. At least 13 different coccidial species are known to infect cattle but not all are pathogenic. The two most pathogenic species of coccidia of cattle in India are *Eimeria bovis* and *E. zuernii* (Deka *et al.*, 1995).

5.5.3. Transmission and pathogenesis

Coccidiosis is transmitted by ingestion of sporulated oocysts. Infection is acquired from contaminated feed, water and soiled pastures or by licking a contaminated hair coat. Coccidia usually infect epithelial cells of the gut mucosa during the developmental stage but in some instances, large, first-generation schizonts of *E. bovis* and *E. zuernii* can be found in endothelial cells of the central lacteals in the small intestine (Hammond *et al.*, 1946) and in connective tissue cells of the lamina propria (Stockdale 1976) respectively.

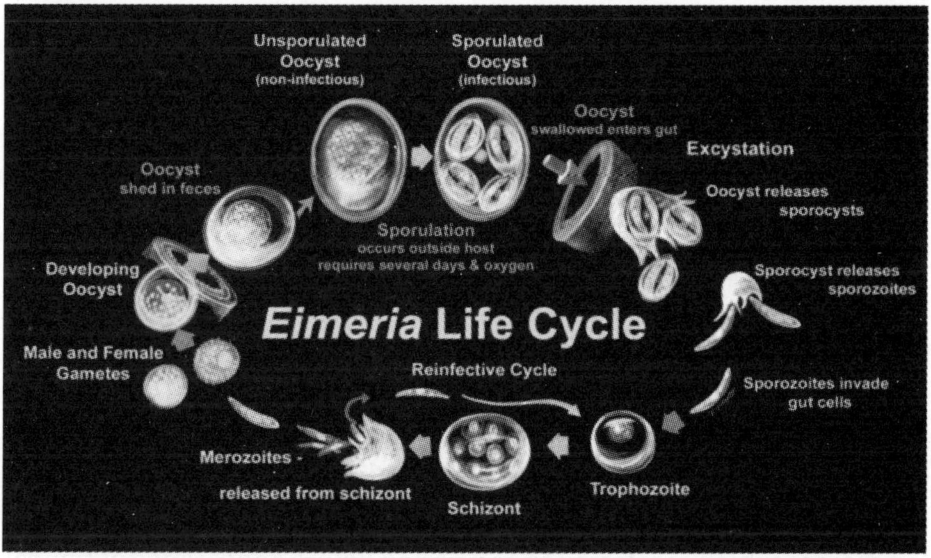

Fig. 24 : Life cycle of *Eimeria* spp. (http://www.en.wikipedia.org)

The clinical course of coccidiosis ranges from 4 to 14 days. Death occurs primarily as a result of diarrhoea, which causes a loss of electrolytes and dehydration. Denatured proteins cause shifts in osmotic pressure, and alter levels of intra- and extra-cellular ions (Roy *et al.*, 1959). Coccidia destroy intestinal cells, which results in loss of blood and other fluids into the small intestine. Blood and other fluid then pass in the feces, which are usually watery. When schizonts are mature, intestinal cells are sloughed from membranes and either leave scattered epithelial cells to cover the lamina propria or expose lamina propria with engorged capillaries (Blaxter and Wood 1958). If these exposed capillaries are severely damaged, blood and plasma may be lost. However, hemorrhaging or secondary complications such as opportunistic infections may contribute to mortality. Animals that recover from severe infections may suffer permanent production losses.

5.5.4. Clinical signs and post mortem findings

Incubation periods for *E. zuernii* and *E. bovis* are usually 15 to 20 days. Immunity to coccidiosis persists only 3 to 4 months and reinfection may occur in the absence of continuous challenge. Signs of the disease include anorexia, loss of weight, and hemorrhagic and mucoid diarrhoea. In severe cases, feces are liquid, bloody and may contain strands of intestinal mucosa. Animals may become emaciated, dehydrated, weak, and listless. Rectal prolapse may result from straining without defecation.

Clinical and subclinical coccidiosis cause economic and health problems for cattle producers. Both forms result in a decline of herd condition mortality can occur, if left untreated. Clinical coccidiosis pertains to responses elicited by the course of the disease. It has been estimated that 5% of infected animals show clinical signs of coccidiosis whether remaining 95% suffer from subclinical form of the disease which is referred to as a period before appearance of typical signs of the disease. This can result in increased economic loss. Since subclinical coccidial infections do not exhibit signs of the disease, animals may get infected without cattle producers knowledge. Losses due to clinical and subclinical coccidiosis result from a decrease in absorption of nutrients due to damage to the intestinal lining (Muirhead 1989).

At necropsy, there may be hemorrhagic enteritis, thickening of mucosa of caecum, colon, rectum and ileum, ulceration and sloughing of intestinal mucosa along with whole blood or blood stained faeces in the lumen of the intestine.

5.5.5. Diagnosis

A presumptive diagnosis of coccidiosis can be made on the basis of clinical signs and post mortem lesions. The basic laboratory diagnostic method depends on the detection of the oocyst of the organism from faecal material. The gene expression profile of sporozoites and first generation merozoites of particularly *E. bovis* can be analyzed by using the technique of differential mRNA display (Abrahamsen *et al.,* 1995). A fluorescence-based technique has also been established to trace intracellular sporozoites of *Eimeria bovis* for tests on gliding motility, invasion, replication and quantification of infection rates in cultured bovine umbilical vein endothelial cells (BUVEC) by laser scanning confocal microscopy and flow cytometry (FCM) analyses and thereby the effect of fluorescent dye 5(6)-carboxyfluorescein diacetate succinimidyl ester (CFSE) on sporozoites at various concentrations and duration of staining can be determined (Hermosilla *et al.,* 2008).

5.5.6. Chemotherapy, prevention and control

For treatment, amprolium (Corid@10mg/kg body wt. for 5 days) is useful whereas lasalocid (Bovatec@1mg/kg/day) and monensin (Rumensin@100-360 mg/kg/day) are the drugs of choice for chemoprophylaxis. Both lasalocid and monensin are polyether ionophores which are used to increase feed efficiency and weight gains apart from preventing coccidiosis (Quigley *et al.,* 1991). Monensin has a lower threshold for toxicity and cattle must be gradually introduced to it in their diet to prevent diarrhoea, feed refusal or toxicity. Other effective preventive measures include minimizing stress by preventing overcrowding, keeping the feed and water at higher level and keeping the shades dry by spreading lime.

5.6. Fascioliasis/ Liver rot

5.6.1. Introduction

Fascioliasis also known as distomatosis/ liver rot is an important helminth disease caused by two trematodes *Fasciola hepatica* (the common liver fluke) and *Fasciola gigantica*. This disease belongs to the plant-borne trematode zoonoses (the zoonotic part will be discussed in Chapter 7). In Europe, the Americas and Oceania only *F. hepatica* is a concern, but the distribution of both species overlap in India (Mascoma *et al.*, 2005). The definitive host range is very broad and includes many herbivorous mammals including cattle.

5.6.2. Etiological agents

Fasciolosis is caused by two digenetic trematodes *F. hepatica* and *F. gigantica*. Adult flukes of both species are localized in the bile ducts of the liver or gallbladder. *F. hepatica* measures 2 to 3 cm and has a cosmopolitan distribution. *F. gigantica* measures 4 to 10 cm in length and the distribution of the species is limited to the tropics (Torgerson and Claxton 1999).

5.6.3. Epidemiology and transmission

Snails from family *Lymnaeidae* act as intermediate host of both *F. hepatica* and *F. gigantica* (Graczyk and Fried 1999) whereas snails from family *Planorbidae* act as an intermediate host of only *F. hepatica*. *Lymnaea rufescens* and *Lymnaea acuminata* are the major host snails in the Indian subcontinent. There are many ecological factors affecting snail populations that include temperature, light, hydrogen ion concentration (pH), vegetation, depth of water, current of the water, chemical composition of the soil and snail population competition.

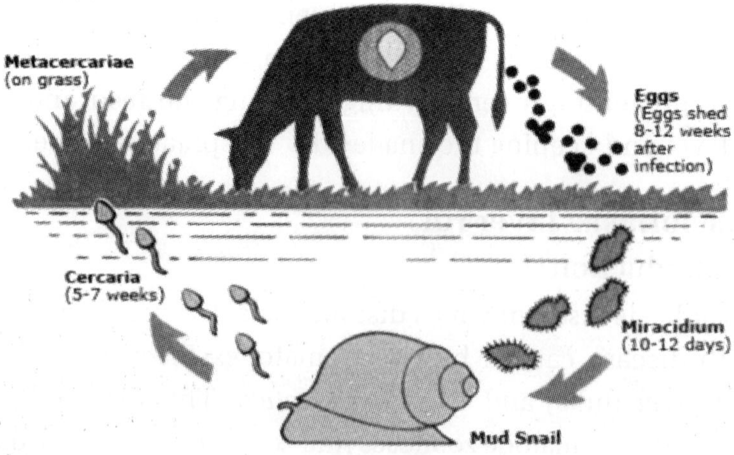

Fig. 25 : Life cycle of *Fasciola* spp. http://www.uk.merial.com.

5.6.4. Pathogenesis

The development of infection in definitive host is divided into two phases: the parenchymal (migratory) phase and the biliary phase (Dubinsky 1993). The parenchymal phase begins when excysted juvenile flukes penetrate the intestinal wall. After the penetration of the intestine, flukes migrate within the abdominal cavity and penetrate the liver or other organs. *F. hepatica* has a strong predilection for the tissues of the liver (Behm and Sangster 1999). Occasionally, ectopic locations of flukes such as the lungs, diaphragm, intestinal wall, kidneys, and subcutaneous tissue can occur (Chen and Mott 1990). During the migration of flukes, tissues are mechanically destroyed and inflammation appears around migratory tracks of flukes. The second phase, known as the biliary phase, begins when parasites enter the biliary ducts of the liver. In biliary ducts, flukes mature, feed on blood and produce eggs. Hypertrophy of biliar ducts associated with obstruction of the lumen occurs as a result of tissue damage. It has been established that cattle acquire resistance to challenge infection with *F. hepatica* and *F. gigantica* when they have been sensitized with primary patent or drug-abbreviated infection (Haroun and Hillyer 1986).

5.6.5. Clinical signs and post mortem lesions

The infection may run acute, subacute or chronic course. In acute case, there may be weakness, ascites, abdominal haemorrhage, icterus and pallor of membrane. In subacute form, drastic weight loss is a predominant feature whereas in chronic cases, the disease may be either asymptomatic or there may be gradual development of bottle jaw, ascites, emaciation and weight loss. In blood, anemia, hypoalbuminemia, and eosinophilia may be observed in all types of fasciolosis. Elevation of liver enzyme activities, such a glutamate dehydrogenase (GLDH), gamma-glutamyl transferase (GGT), and lactate dehydrogenase (LDH), is detected in subacute or chronic fasciolosis from 12-15 week after ingestion of metacercariae (Sykes *et al.*, 1980). However, acquired resistance to *F. hepatica* infection is well known in adult cattle.

At necropsy, during acute phase, the liver is often found damaged badly, swollen and capsule shows many small perforations. Sub capsular haemorrhages and friable liver parenchyma due to tracts of damaged tissues are also characteristic. In chronic cases, there may be presence of large leaf like flukes in grossly enlarged and thicken bile duct. There may be blockage of the bile duct due to presence of flukes and cellular debris. Along with this, there may be extensive fibrosis and calcification of the liver parenchyma.

5.6.6. Diagnosis

Diagnosis of fasciolosis is usually achieved parasitologically by finding the fluke eggs in stool and immunologically by ELISA and Western blot. Coprological examination of faeces is alone not sufficient because eggs of *F. hepatica*, *F. gigantica* and some other trematode like *Fasciolopsis buski* are morphologically indistinguishable (Hillyer 1988). Therefore, immunonological methods such as ELISA and enzyme-linked immunoelectrotransfer blot, also called Western blot, are the most important methods for diagnosis of fascioliasis. These immunological tests are based on detection of species-specific antibodies from sera. The antigenic preparations used have been primarily derived from extracts of excretory/secretory products from adult worms, or with partially purified fractions (Hillyer 1999). Recently, purified native recombinant *F. hepatica* cathepsin L-like protease has also been used (O'Neill *et al.*, 1998). Ultrasonography of the abdominal cavity, biopsy of liver, and gallbladder punctuate also can aid to the diagnosis.

5.6.7. Chemotherapy, prevention and control

Oxyclozanide (Distodin@10-15mg/kg body wt. orally), nitroxynil (Inj. Trodex@10mg/kg body wt. s/c) and supportive therapy of liver extract and vitamin B-comlex are effective.

Since, aquatic snails play an important role in the life cycle of the parasite, thus control of snails by the application of molluscicide is important. The animals should be stall fed and grazing in marshy areas, banks of rivers and ponds should be avoided. Along with this, proper chemoprophylactic treatment of the animal with appropriate flukicide just at the onset of rain is also important.

References

1. Holmes, P.H. (1980) Vaccination against Trypanosomes. *In:* Vaccines against parasites. 1st Edn, eds. Taylor, A. E. R. and Muller, R. Blackwell and Scientific Publications, Oxford, U.K., pp.74-105.
2. Aulakh, G. S. (2003) Haemato-biochemical and therapeutic studies on haemoprotists in bovines. M.V.Sc. thesis, Punjab Agricultural University, Ludhiana, India.
3. http://www.tolweb.org
4. Sumba, A. L., Mihok, S. and Oyieke, F. A (1998). Mechanical transmission of *Trypanosoma evansi* and *T. congolense* by *Stomoxys niger* and *S. taeniatus* in a laboratory mouse model. *Med. Vet. Entomol.*, 12: 417-422.
5. Sridhar, R. K. and Sharma, R. D. (1989) Note on an attempt to transmit *T. evansi* infection through ticks *(Hyalomma anatolicum anatolicum)* in rabbit. *Ind. J. Anim. Hlth.*, 28: 173-174.
6. Juyal, P. D., Singla, L. D. and Saxena, H. M. (1998). *In vivo* activity of human serum against *Trypanosoma evansi* in Swiss albino mice. *J. Parasitic Dis.*, 22: 67-68.
7. Walia, P. S., Kalra, I. S., Juyal, P. D., Sood, N. and Ahuja, S. P. (1996). Role of sialidase activity of *Trypanosoma evansi* in inducing anaemia and immunomodulation in buffalo calves *(Bubalus bubalis)*. *J. Vet. Parasitol.*, 10: 1-9.
8. Touratier, L. (1996). Office International Epizootes. Annual report of a meeting of Adhoc Group on NTTAT (Non-Tse Tse transmitted trypanosomes), France, pp. 2.
9. Juyal, P. D. and Tiwari, H. C. (1982) Effect of cortisone, whole body irradiation and splenectomy on the course of *Trypanosoma evansi* infection in rats. *Ann. Sclavo.*, 24: 523-27.

10. Singla, L. D., Juyal, P. D., Sharma, N. S. and Singh, A. (2001). Responses to haemorrhagic septicaemia vaccination in *Trypanosoma evansi* infected buffalo-calves. Proc. 10th Int. Conf. AITVM (August 20-23), Copenhagen, Denmark.

11. Gupta, M. P., Singla, L. D., Singh, K. B., Mohan, R., Bal, M. S. and Sharma, D. R. (2003). Recrudescence of trypanosomosis following administration of Dexamethasone in bovines. *Ind. Vet. J.*, 80: 360-361.

12. Reid, S. A., Husein, A. and Copeman, D. B. (2001) Evaluation and improvement of parasitological tests for *Trypanosoma evansi* infection. *Vet. Parasitol.*, 102: 291-297.

13. Pathak, K. M. L., Singh,Y., Meiryenne, N. V.and Kapoor, M. (1997) Evaluation of various diagnostic techniques for *Trypanosoma evansi* infections in naturally infected camels. *Vet Parasitol.*, 69: 49-54.

14. Dhami, D. S., Juyal, P. D. and Singla, L. D. (1999). Seroepidemiology of *Trypanosoma evansi* infection using CATT. *Ind. Vet. J.*, 176: 842-844.

15. Omnawar S., Rao, J. R., Singh, R. K. and Butchaiah, G. (2001) DNA amplification in *Trypanosoma evansi* isolates defined by random amplified polymorphic DNA-PCR. *Vet. Rec.*, 148: 244-246.

16. Gill, B. S. (1991). Trypanosomes and trypanosomiases in Indian livestock. ICAR Publication, New Delhi, pp. 2-12.

17. Kaur, P. (2001). Therapeutic effect and kinetic pattern of diminazene aceturate alongwith antipyrine and procaine in experimental typanosomosis in cow-calves. M.V.Sc. thesis, Punjab Agricultural University, Ludhiana, India.

18. Singla, L. D., Juyal, P. D. and Ahuja, S. P. (1998) Blood brain barrier status in experimental *Trypanosoma evansi* infected and levamisole treated cow-calves. *Ind. Vet. J.* 75: 109-112.

19. Singla, L. D. and Juyal, P. D. (1992) Immunomodulatory effects of levamisole against *Trypanosoma evansi* infection in cow-calves: serum gamma globulins. *J. Vet. Parasitol.*, 6: 9-14.

20. Balasubramaniam, G. A. (2004). Pathology of haermoprotozoan diseases in livestock and poultry. *In*: Compendium of summer school on current trends and strategies in diagnosis and control of parasitic diseases of domestic animals and poultry held at Veterinary College, Namakkal from 25 Aug. - 14 Sept. 2004. pp. 135-139.

21. Allsopp, M. T., Cavalier-Smith, T., De Waal, D. T. and Allsopp, B. A. (1994). Phylogeny and evolution of the piroplasms. *Parasitol.,* 108: 147–152.

22. Callow, L. L., Parker, R. J., Rodwell, B. J. and Ottley, M. L. (1976). Piroplasmosis in buffaloes and its serological diagnosis based on a homology between buffalo and bovine immunoglobulins. *Australian Vet. J.*, 52: 40-41.

23. Brown, C. G. D. (1997). Dynamics and impact of tick borne diseases of cattle. *Trop. Anim. Hlth. Prod.*, 29: 1S-3S.

24. http://www.theileria.org.gif.

25. Barnett, S. F. (1977). *Thelieria. In*: Parasitic Protozoa. By Kreier, J. P. Vol IV. Academic Press, New York San Francisco. London.

26. Jithendran, K. P. (2000). A brief profile of blood protista of domestic animals in Himachal Pradesh. *Himachal Vet. J.*, 4: 19-21.

27. Das, G. and D. Ray. (2003). PCR based detection of *Theileria annulata* infection in ticks collected from cattle of West Bengal, India. *J. Vet. Parasitol.*, 17(1): 11-14.

28. Jithendran, K. P. (1997). Blood protista of cattle and buffaloes in Kangra valley, Himachal Pradesh. *Ind. J. Anim. Sci.*, 67: 207-208.

29. Bhikane, A. U., Narladkar, B. W., Anantwar, L. G. and Bhokre, A. P. (2001). Epidemiology, Clinico-pathology and treatment of Babesiosis in Cattle. *Ind. Vet. J.*, 78: 726-729.

30. Bock, R., Jackson, L., De Vos, A. and Jorgensen, W. (2004). Babesiosis of cattle. *Parasitol.*, 129: S247-S269.

31. Mc Leod, R. and Kristjanson, P. (1999). Final report of joint esys/ILRI/ ACIAR TickCost project – Economic impact of ticks and tick-borne diseases to livestock in Africa, Asia and Australia. International Livestock Research Institute, Nairobi.

32. http://www.tulane.edu.gif.

33. Garg, R., Banerjee, P. S., Yadav, C. L. and Garg, A. (2004). Sub clinical Babesiosis and anaplasmosis in crossbred cattle in an organized farm. *J. Vet. Parasitol.*, 18(2): 151-153.

34. Prasad, K. D. (1989). *Babesia* and Babesiosis affecting Indian cattle. *In*: compendium of summer institute on Arthropod borne diseases of domestic animals and birds and their control held at Veterinary college, Ranchi from May 22 - June 10, 1989. pp. 79-88.

35. Sibinovic, K. H., Milar, R., Ristic, M. and Cox, H. W. (1969). In vivo and in vitro effects of serum antigens of parasitized and normal erythrocytes. *Ann. Trop. Med. Parasit.*, 63: 327-336.

36. Mahoney, D. F. (1977). *Babesia* in domestic animals. *In*: Parasitic protozoa, vol. 4, Kreier, J. P. (Ed). Academic press, New York, pp. 1-52.

37. Shastri, L. V. and Kulkarni, G. B. (1988). Second National Congress of Veterinary Parasitology. pp. 16-17.

38. Lohr, K. F. (1973). Susceptibility of non-splenectomized and splenectomized Sahiwal cattle to experimental *Babesia bigemina* infection. *Zentralblatt fu¨r Veterinarmedizin Reihe.*, [B] 20: 52–56.

39. Dalgliesh, R. J. (1993). Babesiosis. In Immunology and Molecular Biology of Parasite Infections (ed. Warren, S. K.), pp. 352–383. Oxford, Blackwell.

40. Smith, R. D., Molinar, E., Larios, F., Monroy, J., Trigo, F. and Ristic, M. (1980). Bovine babesiosis: pathogenicity and heterologous species immunity of tick-borne *Babesia bovis* and *B. bigemina* infections. *Am. J. Vet. Res.*, 41: 1957–1965.

41. Wright, I. G., Goodger, B. V., Leatch, G., Aylward, J. H., Rode-Bramanis, K. and Waltisbuhl, D. J. (1987). Protection of *Babesia bigemina*-immune animals against subsequent challenge with virulent *Babesia bovis*. *Infect. Immun.*, 55: 364–368.

42. Potgieter, F. T. (1977). The life cycle of *Babesia bovis* and *Babesia bigemina* in ticks and in cattle in South Africa. PhD thesis, Rand Afrikaans University.

43. De Vos, A. J. and Potgieter, F. T. (1994). Bovine babesiosis. In Infectious Diseases of Livestock (ed. Coetzer, J. A. W., Thomson, G. R. and Tustin, R. C.), pp. 278–294. Capetown, Oxford University Press.

44. Johnston, L. A., Trueman, K. F. and Pearson, R. D. (1977). Bovine babesiosis: comparison of fluorescent antibody and giemsa staining in post-mortem diagnosis of infeciton. *Australian Vet. J.*, 53: 222–226.

45. Harkirat, S., Mishra, A. K., Rao, J. R. and Tewari, A. K. (2007). Seroprevalence of babesiosis in cattle and buffaloes by indirect fluorescent antibody test. *J. Vet. Parasitol.*, 21(1): 1-4.

46. Böse, R., Jorgensen, W. K., Dalgliesh, R. J., Friedhoff, K. T. and De Vos, A. J. (1995). Current state and future trends in the diagnosis of babesiosis. *Vet. Parasitol.*, 57: 61–74.

47. Ravindran, R., Mishra, A. K. and Rao, J. R. (2008). Randomly amplified polymorphic DNA-polymerase chain reaction fingerprinting of *Babesia bigemina* isolates of India. *Veterinarski Archiv.*, 78(6): 545-551.

48. De Vos, A. J. (1979). Epidemiology and control of bovine babesiosis in South Africa. *J. South African Vet. Assoc.*, 50: 357–362.

49. Taylor, R. J. and Mc Hardy, N. (1979). Preliminary observations on the combined use of imidocarb and Babesia blood vaccine in cattle. *J. South African Vet. Assoc.*, 50: 326–329.

50. Perry, B. D., Chamboko, T., Mahan, S. M., Medley, G. F., Minjauw, B., O'Callaghan, C. J. and Peter, T. F. (1998). The economics of integrated tick and tick borne disease control on commercial farms in Zimbabwe. Zimbabwe. *Vet. J.*, 29: 21–29.

51. Callow, L. L. and Dalgliesh, R. J. (1980). The development of effective, safe vaccination against babesiosis and anaplasmosis in Australia. *In*: Ticks and Tick-borne Diseases. Proceedings of a Symposium held at the 56th Annual Conference of the Australian Veterinary Association (ed. Johnston, L. A. Y. and Cooper, M. G.), pp. 4–8. Townsville, Australian Veterinary Association.

52. Norimine, J., Suarez, C. E., Mc Elwain, T. F., Florin-Christensen, M. and Brown, W. C. (2002). Immunodominant epitopes in Babesia bovis rhoptry-associated protein 1 that elicit memory CD4(+)-T-lymphocyte responses in B. bovis-immune individuals are located in the amino-terminal domain. *Infect. Immun.*, 70: 2039–2048.

53. Fitzgerald, P. R. (1975). The significance of bovine coccidiosis as a disease in the United States. *Bovine Pract.*, 10: 28.

54. Ernst, J. V. and Benz, G. W. (1986). Intestinal coccidiosis in cattle. The veterinary clinics of North America/parasites: epidemiology and control. W.B. Saunders Company, Philadelphia, PA.

55. Deka, D. K., Choudhury, S. and Choudhury, A. (1995). Parasites of domestic animals and birds in Likhimpur (Assam). *J. Vet. Parasitol.*, 9(1): 21-25.

56. Hammond, M., G. W., Bowman, L. R. D. and Simms, B. T. (1946). The endogenous phase of the life cycle of Eimeria bovis. *J. Parasit.*, 32: 409.

57. Stockdale, P. G. (1976). Schizogony and gametogony of *Eimeria zuernii* (Rivolta, 1878) Martin, 1909. *Vet. Parasit.*, 1: 367.

58. http://www.en.wikipedia.org.

59. Roy, J. B., Hawkins, K. W., Gillian, H., Lang, J. M. and Ingraham, P. L. (1959). The effect of white scours on the sodium and potassium concentration in the serum of newborn calves. *Br. J. Nutr.*, 13: 219.

60. Blaxter, K. L. and Wood, W. A. (1958). Some observations on the biochemical events associated with diarrhea in calves. *Vet. Rec.*, 65: 889.

61. Muirhead, S. (1989). Coccidiosis infections often go undetected in beef, dairy cattle. *Feedstuffs.*, 15: 87.

62. Abrahamsen, M. S., Johnson, R. R., Hathaway, M. and White, M. W. (1995). Identification of Eimeria bovis merozoite cDNAs using differential mRNA display. *Mol. Biochem. Parasitol.*, 71(2): 183-191.

63. Hermosilla, C., Stamm, I., Taubert, A., Lutz, K., Zahner, H. and Menge, C. (2008). Fluorecent Eimeria bovis sporozoites and meront stages in vitro: a helpful tool to study parasite-host cell interactions. *Parasitol. Res.*, 102(4): 777-786.

64. Quigley, J. D., Caldwell, L. A., Sinks, G. D. and Heitmann, R. N. (1991). Blood glucose, nonesterified fatty acids and ketones in response to weaning and feed intake in young calves. *J. Dairy Sci.*, 74: 250.

65. Mas-Coma, S., Bargues, M. D. and Valero, M. A. (2005). Fascioliasis and other plant-borne trematode zoonoses. *Int. J. Parasitol.*, 35 (11–12): 1255–1278.

66. Torgerson, P. and Claxton, J. (1999). Epidemiology and control. *In*: Dalton, J. P. Fasciolosis. Wallingford, Oxon, UK: CABI Pub. pp. 113–149.

67. Graczyk, T. K and Fried, B. (1999). Development of *Fasciola hepatica* in the intermediate host. *In*: Dalton, J. P. Fasciolosis. Wallingford, Oxon, UK: CABI Pub. pp. 31–46.

68. http://www.uk.merial.com.

69. Dubinský, P. (1993). Trematódy a trematodózy. In: Jurášek, V., Dubinský, P. a kolektív, Veterinárna parazitológia. Príroda a. s., Bratislava, 158–187. (in Slovakian).

70. Behm, C. A. and Sangster, N. C. (1999). Pathology, pathophysiology and clinical aspects. *In*: Dalton, J. P. (Ed.), Fasciolosis. CAB International Publishing, Wallingford, pp. 185–224.

71. Chen, M. G. and Mott, K. E. (1990). Progress in assessment of morbidity due to Fasciola hepatica infection: a review of recent literature. *Trop. Dis. Bull.*, 87: R1–R38.

72. Haroun, E. T. and Hillyer, G. V. (1986). Resistance to fascioliasis—a review. *Vet. Parasitol.*, 20(1–3): 63–93.

73. Sykes, A. R., Coop, A. R. and Robinson, M. G. (1980). Chronic subclinical ovine fascioliasis: plasma glutamate dehydrogenase, gamma glutamyl transpeptidase and aspartate aminotransferase activities and their significance as diagnostic aids. *Res. Vet. Sci.*, 28: 71–78.

74. Hillyer, G. V. (1988). Fascioliasis and fasciolopsiasis. *In*: Turano, A., Albert, B. and Ohashi, M. *Laboratory diagnosis of infectious diseases: principles and practices*. Bacterial, mycotic, and parasitic diseases. Berlin: Springer-Verlag. pp. 856–862.

75. Hillyer, G. V. (1999). Immunodiagnosis of human and animal fasciolosis. *In*: Dalton, J. P. *Fasciolosis*. Wallingford, Oxon, UK: CABI Pub. pp. 435–447.

76. O'Neill, S. M., Parkinson, M., Strauss, W., Angles, R. and Dalton, J. P. (1998). Immunodiagnosis of Fasciola hepatica infection (fascioliasis) in a human population in the Bolivian Altiplano using purified cathepsin L cysteine proteinase. *Am. J. Trop. Med. Hyg.*, 58(4): 417–423.

□□□

Chapter 6

Major Infectious Causes of Abortion in Cattle in India

Numerous bacterial, fungal, viral and protozoan pathogens have been associated with infertility and abortion in cattle. These pathogens can result in substantial economic losses, indicating the need for control measures to prevent infection or disease. This chapter deals with the reproductive dysgenesis that compromise viability of domestic animals prior to parturition. Although more deaths occur at and around birth than between 1 week of age and weaning, embryonic losses are usually higher than perinatal losses. Notably, maternal infections during pregnancy may or may not impact fetal development. The impact on fetal development may be caused directly by infectious agents or their toxins, or indirectly by placentitis. Furthermore, detection of a reproductive pathogen should not preclude further diagnostic testing as dual infections are not uncommon.

6.1. Brucellosis

Brucella abortus is a zoonotic, gram-negative coccobacillus, transmitted via ingestion of fetus, placenta, uterine discharge, or materials contaminated by these products. Through hematogenous spread, the bacteria localize in the trophoblasts. Abortions generally occur after the fifth month of gestation (usually between 6-9 months of gestation). Retained fetal membranes and metritis often occur (Barr and Anderson 1993). Incubation period of abortion varies from 2 weeks to 6 months. Apart from abortion, there may be still birth, weak calves, retained placenta, infertility and mastitis. Maternal cotyledons may be necrotic and brownish to dirty yellow (which is time dependent). In fetus, there is no specific finding. Blood-tinged subcutaneous edema and blood- tinged fluid in serous cavities may be frequently found. Abomasal contents may be whitish cloudy yellow to reddish, depending on degree of autolysis. Inerestingly, bronchopneumonia is common. Udder is the site of persistent infection in approximately 50% of infected cows. Low grade chronic interstitial mastitis develops in carrier animals that shed the organisms in milk. Chronic lymphadenitis of supramammary lymph node is characteristic along with hygroma. In bulls, there may be development of painful orchitis, periorchitis, epididymitis and seminal vesiculitis. Diagnosis is based on the detection of organisms in the cotyledonary and fetal abomasal smears by MAF staining and conducting FAT on cotyledons, fetal abomasal contents and tissues. Serum agglutination test (SAT) titre of more than 1:100 in maternal sera is considered as positive. Along with the above techniques, simultaneous cultural examination should be conducted from specimens like fetal abomasums, maternal cotyledons, uterine fluids and milk.

6.2. Leptospirosis

Leptospira spp. are zoonotic spirochetes. Cattle are the maintenance hosts for *Leptospira interrogans* serovar *hardjo* (type hardjoprajitno) and *Leptospira borgpetersenii* serovar *hardjo* (type hardjo-bovis). Transmission among maintenance hosts is through contact with infected urine, milk, placental fluid, transplacentally, or venereally (Yaeger and Holler 2007). Transmission to an incidental host occurs via contact with an environment contaminated with infected urine. The bacteria gain access through the mucous membranes of the eyes, nose, vagina or abraded skin. Infection in pregnant animals can lead to abortion, stillbirth, or birth of weak calves. Abortion caused by serovar *hardjo* occurs from 4 months of gestation to term. Infertility is also considered to occur with serovar *hardjo* infections. The diagnostics include direct FAT conducted on fetus, histopathologic demonstration by special stains culture and direct demonstration of the organisms in maternal urine by darkfield or phase contrast microscopy. However, maternal paired serum samples are of little use as titers are static or falling after abortion.

6.3. Listeriosis

Infection with Listeria monocytogenes occurs through ingestion of the organism in poor-quality alkaline silage or pastures contaminated with feces containing the zoonotic organism (Menzies 2007). Transmission is through ingestion and intestinal carrier state is common in cattle. There are two forms of the diseases *viz.*, neural and genital. Genital listeric infection results in abortion, premature births, stillbirths and neonatal deaths. Abortion may be sporadic or multiple and can reach upto 50%. Abortions usually occur in the last trimester. Usually, there is chronic involvement of the placenta and cotyledonary necrosis is marked. There may be death of the fetus *in utero* along with autolytic changes. Small, pin-point yellow foci of hepatic necrosis measuring about 0.5 - 1.0 mm in diameter and small shallow ulcers in the abomasums and larynx, around 1-2 mm are characteristic. Diagnosis is based on cultural examination of the organisms from specimens like placenta, fetal abomasal contents and lung along with histopathology and FAT conducted on placental tissue and fetus respectively.

6.4. Campylobacteriosis

Campylobacter fetus sub species *venerealis* infection is primarily an infertility inducing disease caising embryonic mortality and is always associated with current infertility history. Transmission is through venereal route. Abortion rate is low and may be less than 10%. Abortions occur at any stage of gestation, usually between 4-7 months. Placental lesions are similar to brucellosis but usually less severe. Maternal cotyledons become necrosed, yellowish and soft (Givens and Marley 2008). Diagnostics include demonstration of the organisms by darkfield microscopy revealing characteristic sea gull appearance of the organisms, phase contrast microscopy on stained smears, FAT to be conducted on placenta and fetal abomasal contents along with vaginal mucus agglutination test (VMAT) on a herd basis. Histopathology may reveal mild fetal pneumonia.

6.5. Salmonellosis

Abortion due to *Salmonella typhimurium* is usually secondary to gastroenteritis. Transmission occurs through ingestion. There is development of oedema in placenta along with autolytic changes. Death of foetus occurs *in utero* due to septicaemia (Report published by Scott, P. in NADIS Health Bulletin). Primary isolation can be carried out in enrichment media like tetrathionate broth or selenite F broth followed by plating in enriched and selective media like Mc Konkey agar, Brilliant Green agar and Salmonella-Shigiella medium ,applying series of biochemical tests like sugar fermentation and acid production (Triple sugar iron test), production of hydrogen sulphide, urease, indole, acetoin, citrate utilization, determining the proteiolytic property by gelatine liquefaction test and growth in KCN medium.

6.6. Mycoplasmal abortion

Ureaplasma diversum and *Mycoplasma* spp. including *M. bovigenitalium* and *M. agalactiae* var bovis are the major pathogens causing abortion in cattle. Although Ureaplasma diversum and *Mycoplasma* spp. are part of the normal flora of the reproductive tract, they can cause reproductive failure (Doig 1981). Trans- mission can occur through direct contact, environmental contamination with infected urine, and venereally. Infection with *U. diversum* can lead to granular vulvitis, infertility, abortion, and birth of weak calves. *Mycoplasma bovigenitalium* infection can cause granular vulvovaginitis, infertility, and endometritis. Experimentally, *Mycoplasma bovis* can cause endometritis, salpingitis, infertility and abortion. However, the role of Mycoplasma in causing abortion in cattle requires further studies.

6.7. Mycotic abortion

Mycotic abortions can be caused by various molds and yeasts (Walker 2007). *Aspergillus fumigatus* is the most common pathogen that accounts for 60-80% of the sporadic abortion caused by fungi. Other pathogens include *Absidia*, *Rhizomucor*, *Rhizopus*, *Penicillium* and *Candida*. The disease occurs sporadically, usually when animals are housed indoors or in small pens and fed hay. It has been observed that less than 5% of the cows in a herd get affected upon exposure to the agent. The fungal pathogens may enter the respiratory or gastrointestinal tract and then gain access to the systemic circulation and spread to the placentomes. Incubation period is commonly 35 days and above. Abortion generally occurs between 6 and 8 months of gestation (Barr and Anderson 1993). Placentitits and retained placenta are frequent occurrences. Lesions are striking. Placentomes are greatly enlarged, reddish to yellow, necrotic with swollen inturned margins, friable centers and firmly incarcerated. Fetis are born either dead or weak and nonviable. One-third of the fetus have characteristic signs of mycotic dermatitis involving the periorbit, eyelids, occuiput, shoulders, back and sides. Areas are slightly raised, grayish, irregular and tend to coalesce. Pneumonia may be found occasionally. Diagnosis is based on detection of fungal morphology by KOH wet mounts and phase contrast microscopy conducted on smears made from edges of cotyledons or placentomes and fetal abomasal contents along with cultural examination and histopathology of the specimen collected from fetal skin. Thrombosis of the placental blood vessels can also be revealed by histopathology.

6.8. Infectious bovine rhinotracheitis (IBR)

Bovine herpesvirus 1 is an alpha herpesvirus that can lead to respiratory and genital infections, as well as abortion (Muylkens *et al.*, 2007). Transmission occurs through contact with upper respiratory, conjunctival or genital tract mucous membranes, aborted fetuses, or through venereal transmission. Abortions are most commonly associated with the respiratory form of the disease and not the genital form. Cows can have fever, anorexia, red nasal mucosa, coughing, and conjunctivitis, followed by abortion in 15–64 days. Abortion generally occurs between 4 and 8 months of gestation and abortion rate varies from 5-60%. Infection also can result in early embryonic death (Miller and Van der Maaten 1986). Bovine herpesvirus 1 establishes latent infections in the trigeminal and sacral ganglia and following immunosuppression, the virus can become reactivated. Therefore, these animals serve as a source of infection for unexposed cattle. Retention of placenta is a common feature of infection and the cotyledons may show blanched necrotic appearance. Fetuses usually die 24-48 hours before expulsion and there may be variable degree of autolysis, blood-tinged subcutaneous oedema and fluid accumulation in the serous cavities. Along with these, there may be autolytic changes in the kidney, small necrotic foci of around 0.2-0.5 mm in liver, lymph nodes, spleen and adrenals. Diagnosis can be made on the basis of demonstration of intranuclear inclusions in histopathological section of foetal lungs, testes and liver along with demonstration of viral antigen in the section of kidney cotyledons by FAT. 2-4 fold increase in maternal antibody titre is indicative of IBR.

6.9. Trichomoniasis

Tritrichomonas foetus is a flagellated protozoa that causes venereal disease in cattle (Peter 1997). Infected cows can experience early embryonic death, infertility, and abortion in the first half of gestation. Some cows develop postcoital pyometra. Recent experimental evidence indicates that the fetus is not attacked by the trichomonads until approximately day 50 of gestation. Fetal loss usually occurs 2 to 5 months following infected service. However, the abortion rate is low and usually occurs in the first half of gestation and rarely after the 5th month. Placental and fetal lesions are non-specific and often not observed. Diagnosis is mainly dependent on the direct demonstration and culturing of trichomonads in the placental fluid, fetal abomasal contents and vaginal discharge and demonstration of the characteristic motility.

References

1. Barr, B. C. and Anderson, M. L. (1993). Infectious diseases causing bovineabortion and fetal loss. *Vet. Clin. North Am. Food Anim. Pract.*, 9: 343–368.

2. Yaeger, M. J. and Holler, L. D. (2007). Bacterial causes of bovine infertility and abortion. *In*: Youngquist RS, Threlfall WR, editors. Current therapy in large animal theriogenology. 2nd ed., St. Louis: Elsevier. pp. 389–399.

3. Menzies, P. A. (2007). Abortion in sheep: diagnosis and control. *In*: Youngquist, R. S. and Threlfall, W. R. editors. Current therapy in large animal theriogenology. 2nd ed., St. Louis: Elsevier. pp. 667–680.

4. Givens, D. and Marley, M. S. D. (2008). Infectious causes of embryonic and fetal mortality. *Theriogenol.*, doi:10.1016/j.theriogenology.2008.04.018.

5. Scott, P. *In*: NADIS Health Bulletin.

6. Doig, P. A. (1981). Bovine genital mycoplasmosis. *Can. Vet. J.*, 22: 339–343.

7. Walker, R. L. (2007). Mycotic bovine abortion. *In*: Youngquist, R. S. and Threlfall, W. R. editors. Current therapy in large animal theriogenology. 2nd ed., St. Louis: Elsevier. pp. 417–419.

8. Barr, B. C. and Anderson, M. L. (1993). Infectious diseases causing bovine abortion and fetal loss. *Vet. Clin. North Am. Food Anim. Pract.*, 9: 343–368.

9. Muylkens, B., Thiry, J., Kirten, P., Schynts, F. and Thiry, E. (2007). Bovine herpesvirus 1 infection and infectious bovine rhinotracheitis. *Vet. Res.*, 38: 181–209.

10. Miller, J. M, Van Der Maaten, M. J. (1986). Experimentally induced infectious bovine rhinotracheitis virus infection during early pregnancy: effect on the bovine corpus luteum and conceptus. *Am. J. Vet. Res.*, 47: 223–228.

11. Peter, D. (1997). Bovine venereal diseases. *In*: Youngquist, R. S. editor. Current therapy in large animal theriogenology. Philadelphia: W.B. Saunders Co., pp. 355–363.

❑❑❑

Chapter 7

Major Infectious Diseases of Cattle Having Public Health Concern

Changes in pathogen and host ecology are primarily responsible for the majority of diseases transmissible to human. Ecological changes embrace a number of processes under the same umbrella *viz.*, changes in agricultural practices, urbanisation, globalisation or climate change (Schrag and Wiener 1995). Factors associated with the emergence of pathogens in human and domestic animals like cattle have been explored from time to time (Daszak *et al.*, 2001). In recent years, it seems that humans have probably been responsible for many zoonotic diseases through creating and maintaining the conditions for existing pathogens to enter, persist and develop in new host populations (Dobson and Foufopulos 2001). Disease emergence is the result of two sequential processes *viz.*, the adaptation of a pathogen to a new host and the spread of the pathogen into the new population. These pathogens have adverse effects on indigenous fauna and are considered to be one of the most important causes of the global biodiversity crisis. They are also recognised as a clear threat to ecosystems, habitats or species, with severe economic and environmental consequences (CBD 2003). Such pathogens are of great public health concern and the diseases caused by them may be acquired or spread in a variety of ways *viz.*, through the air (aerosol), by direct contact, by contact with an inanimate object that harbors the disease (fomite transmission), by oral ingestion, and by insect transmission. The present chapter gives a brief outline of such diseases.

7.1. Anthrax

Anthrax is a naturally occurring disease with worldwide distribution. It is caused by *Bacillus anthracis*, a spore-forming bacteria that can remain dormant in the soil for many years. The organism can bloom and contaminate surface soil and grass after periods of wet, cool weather, followed by several weeks of hot, dry conditions. The anthrax zones are found in areas wherein the soil is heavily contaminated with anthrax spores. Such conditions include soil rich in organic matter (pH <6.0) and dramatic changes in climate, such as abundant rainfall following a prolonged drought. Anthrax can infect humans in three ways which have been discussed in chapter 1 and so also will be discussed now. Skin anthrax also known as the cutaneous anthrax may be contracted by handling contaminated hair, wool, hides, flesh, blood, or feces of infected animals, as well as through manufactured products such as bone meal. Infection is introduced through scratches, abrasions, or wounds of the skin. It is the mildest form of human anthrax. Symptoms include itching, rash and lesions near the site of infection. With proper treatment, skin anthrax is fatal in less than 1% of all cases. Approximately 95% of human anthrax infections are cutaneous infections. Gastrointestinal anthrax is contracted by orally ingesting anthrax spores, usually by eating insufficiently cooked infected meat. Symptoms include cramps, diarrhoea, and fever. Gastrointestinal anthrax infections are unlikely from handling contaminated packages. Inhalation anthrax is contracted by inhaling spores directly into the lungs. Such infections normally occur among workers handling infected animal hides. After an incubation period of one to seven days, the infected individual gradually develops flu-like symptoms such as fever, malaise, fatigue, cough, and mild chest discomfort. This mild disease can progress rapidly to respiratory distress and shock in two to four days, followed by a range of more severe symptoms such as difficulty in breathing and exhaustion. Under natural conditions, inhaled anthrax is exceedingly rare (Friedlander 1999). In case of human anthrax, post exposure prophylaxis may be achieved with oral ciprofloxacin (500 mg twice a day) or doxycycline (100 mg twice a day). Biothrax vaccine has been developed in USA which is an alum precipitated toxoid containing protective antigen treated with formalin. Chemoprophylaxis is best continued until the exposed person has received at least three doses of vaccine for a minimum period of 4 weeks). If vaccine is unavailable, chemoprophylaxis has to be continued for 8 weeks (Friedlanders *et al.,* 1993).

7.2. Brucellosis

Brucella organisms can be present in birthing tissues or fluids (aborted fetuses, fetal fluids, placentas, and vaginal discharges), and also in milk, urine, blood, and semen. Transmission among cattle is through ingestion of birthing fluids and milk and *in utero*. Most infections in humans are associated with drinking or eating unpasteurized milk products. Much of the milk which is consumed is rendered safe by pasteurisation or boiling, but cheese is preferably prepared from untreated milk. During the course of cheese manufacture, any *Brucella* present in the milk become trapped in the clot and thus concentrated in the cheese, although bacteria may subsequently be inactivated by manufacturing or ripening processes. Cream and ice cream prepared from milk also possess risk of transmission (Flores-Castro and Baer 1980). Handling infected aborted fetuses or afterbirth is another common means of human infection due to the entry of the organisms through cuts in the skin and the mucous membranes of the eye and mouth.

Common symptoms in humans are undulating fever, weakness, headache, joint pain along with night sweats. Human brucellosis can be prevented by avoiding drinking of unpasteurised/untreated dairy products and wearing gloves when handling reproductive tissues. Hands should be washed after touching or handling animals.

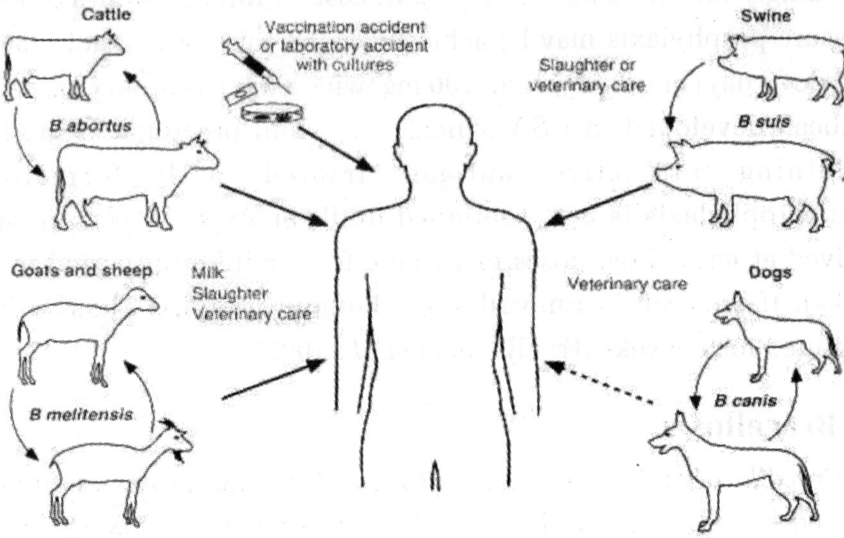

Fig. 26 : Transmission of different species of *Brucella* including *B. abortus* from animals to human (This material is the property of Live care Foundation)

7.3. *Escherichia coli* infection

Escherichia coli (*E. coli)* are bacteria normally found in the intestines of human and cattle. However, some strains cause a severe, often bloody, diarrhea in humans. Cattle act as the carriers of the bacteria and humans become infected by ingesting contaminated food or water, especially undercooked groun beef (Bielaszewska *et al.*, 1997). Humans may also become infected after handling or being exposed to feces of a carrier animal. Person-to-person transmission can occur by lack of good hand washing following diaper changes. *E. coli* O157: H7 is a particularly virulent strain of *E. coli* that causes asymptomatic infection in cattle in most of the instances but has the potential of causing abdominal cramping and bloody diarrhea in human occasionally life threatening kidney disease and a hemolytic uremic syndrome in children and elderly person. Prevention focuses on hand washing and proper food hygiene. Hands and all cooking equipment should be washed with soap and hot water after touching or handling raw meat. Meats should be thawed in the refrigerator, and ground beef should be cooked until it reaches an internal temperature of 165°F and the juices run clear. Eating undercooked meat or drinking unpasteurised milk should be avoided. Hands should be washed after handling animals and eating or drinking around animals should be avoided. Day-care facilities should wash toys frequently, and individuals with diarrhea should avoid swimming in public areas. In outbreaks of other primary transmission routes, secondary cases occur, which emphasizes the importance of educating caretakers to avoid direct contact with faecal matter and to apply stringent hand washing rules. Virulent O157 antigen-specific phages can play a role in effective biocontrol of the infection in animals and fresh food stuffs without compromising the viability of other normal flora or food quality (Kudva *et al.*, 1999).

7.4. Salmonellosis

Salmonella spp. are shed in the feces of infected animals. Many animals are susceptible to *Salmonella* including cattle. Infection occurs as a result of the ingestion of contaminated feed, water, or grass. The bacterium can live for months to years in the environment, especially in wet and warm conditions. People acquire *Salmonella* from undercooked contaminated meat or unpasteurized milk products. If hands are not washed after direct contact with infected feces, then accidental ingestion of bacteria can occur. Humans may develop diarrhea, abdominal cramping and fever which can be very severe. For primary screening of human cases (especially paratyphoid caused by *S. paratyphi*), Widal test is most frequently employed which is a slide agglutination test for detecting somatic A and B antigens followed by detection of flagellar H antigen. Drugs like chloramphenicol and imepenam are used for treatment of human infection but there is chance of multiple drug resistance and thus the antibiogram profiles needed to be studied first. Regular microbiological monitoring of the slaughter house by products, insect control, preventing the pet animals from consuming inedible offals are among some of the basic preventive measures. Meat should be adequately cooked and proper food handling hygiene should be used. Hands should always be washed after touching or working with animals. Strategies for preventing infection by raw milk cheeses should be aimed at both producers and consumers. Strict and carefully planned hazard analysis critical control point procedures should be developed and implemented for unpasteurised dairy products (Robinson and Jones 1981). As part of this procedure any batch of cheese made from raw milk should be closely monitored for *Salmonella* and distribution should be avoided until known to be clear. Producers should also report positive results of end production internal sampling to public health authorities. Consumers particularly those susceptible to infectious diseases (*eg.,* infants, elderly people and immunocompromised patients) should also be warned that a nil risk cannot be warranted for raw milk products.

7.5. Tuberculosis (T.B)

Humans may acquire *M. bovis,* the causative agent of bovine tuberculosis from unpasteurized dairy products and can develop symptoms involving the lungs, kidneys, spine, or brain. Infected individuals have a persistent cough and often cough up blood. There is increasing need of screening human patients for T.B by performing Mantoux test which is an intradermal skin test that detects skin thickness of 5 mm or more 48-72 hours following the administration of liquid tuberculin. Several drugs like streptomycin, para-amino-salicilic acid, isoniazid and rifampicin are available for treatment of T.B in human. The cornerstone of treatment for TB lies in the use of combination of drugs like isoniazid, rifampicin, pyrazinamide and ethambutol for two months followed by isoniazid and rifampicin alone for a further four months. The patient is considered cured at six months, even though there is still a relapse rate of 2 to 3%. For latent tuberculosis, the standard treatment is six to nine months of isoniazid alone (Grange and Zumla 2002). Prevention is by avoiding consumption of unpasteurized dairy products.

7.6. Leptospirosis

Leptospirosis is a zoonoses which can be transmitted from animal to animal and animal to human. The original natural carrier for serovar *icterohaemorrhagiae* is rodent. Cattle acts as the rervoir host for Lepto serovar *hardjo-bovis*. Transmission of the organism to human can occur through skin abrasions and mucous membranes by contact with urine or tissues of animals infected with leptospirosis. Apart from this, ingestion and inhalation can also transmit the disease. Human infections vary from asymptomatic to severe. Many cases are mild or asymptomatic and remain unrecognized. Usually, it occurs as a biphasic illness in human. The first phase, called the acute or septicemic phase begins abruptly and lasts approximately a week. This phase is characterized by nonspecific signs including fever, chills, headache and conjunctival suffusion. Myalgia, which typically affects the back, thighs or calves, is often severe. Occasionally, a transient skin rash occurs. Other symptoms may include weakness, photophobia, lymphadenopathy, abdominal pain, nausea, vomiting, a sore throat, cough, chest pain and hemoptysis. Mental confusion, neck stiffness and other signs of aseptic meningitis are also characteristics of this phase. Jaundice can be seen in more severe infections. These symptoms last for approximately 4 to 9 days, then are typically followed by a 1 to 3 day period during which the temperature drops and the symptoms disappear. The second phase of leptospirosis, called the immune phase, is characterized by the development of anti-*Leptospira* antibodies, and the excretion of the organisms in the urine. This phase can last up to 30 days or more, but does not develop in all patients. During the immune phase, the patient becomes ill again. Nonspecific fever and myalgia are seen during the first phase recur but may be less severe than in the first stage of disease. Two forms of disease, icteric and anicteric, are seen. Most infections are of the anicteric form. The most important symptoms in this form are associated with aseptic meningitis. A severe headache, stiff neck and other meningeal symptoms occur in approximately half of all patients, and usually last a few days. Occasionally, these signs may be present for up to two weeks. Less common symptoms include cranial nerve paralysis, encephalitis, confusion and changes in consciousness. Deaths are rare in the typical anicteric form. However, a syndrome of fatal pulmonary hemorrhage, without jaundice, has recently been reported. The icteric form is more severe. It occurs in 5-10% of all patients, is often rapidly progressive, and may be associated with multiorgan failure. The most commonly involved organ systems are the liver, kidneys and central nervous system (CNS). In the icteric form, there may be no period of improvement between the septicemic and immune phases. Jaundice can be severe and may give the skin an orange tone, but it is not usually associated with severe hepatic necrosis. Acute renal failure occurs in 16-40% of cases (OIE 2005). Some patients also have pulmonary symptoms, with clinical signs ranging from cough, dyspnea, chest pain, and mild to severe hemoptysis, to adult respiratory distress syndrome. Cardiac involvement can result in congestive heart failure, myocarditis and pericarditis. Hemorrhages may also be seen; epistaxis, petechiae, purpura and ecchymoses are the most common signs, but severe gastrointestinal bleeding, adrenal or subarachnoid hemorrhage, and pulmonary hemorrhages can occur. Rare complications include stroke, rhabdomyolysis, thrombotic thrombocytopenic purpura, acute acalculous cholecystitis, erythema nodosum, aortic stenosis, Kawasaki syndrome, reactive arthritis, epididymitis, nerve palsy, male hypogonadism, Guillain-Barre´ syndrome and cerebral arteritis. Deaths can occur from kidney failure, cardiac involvement. pulmonary hemorrhage or other serious organ dysfunction. Convalescence from the icteric form may take 1-2 months. Although jaundice can persist for weeks, liver function returns to normal after recovery, and hepatic disease is rarely the cause of death. Most patients also recover kidney function. Anterior uveitis occurs up to a year after recovery. Iridocyclitis and chorioretinitis can also be complications, and may persist for years. Abortions, fetal death, and rare congenital infections in newborns are among the problems associated with reproductive failure. Abortions can occur at any time, including the convalescent period. As far as the human to human transmission is concerned, it occurs rarely. *Leptospira* organisms are found in the urine during the second (immune) phase of the disease. Most people excrete these bacteria for 60 days or less, but shedding for months or years have also been documented.

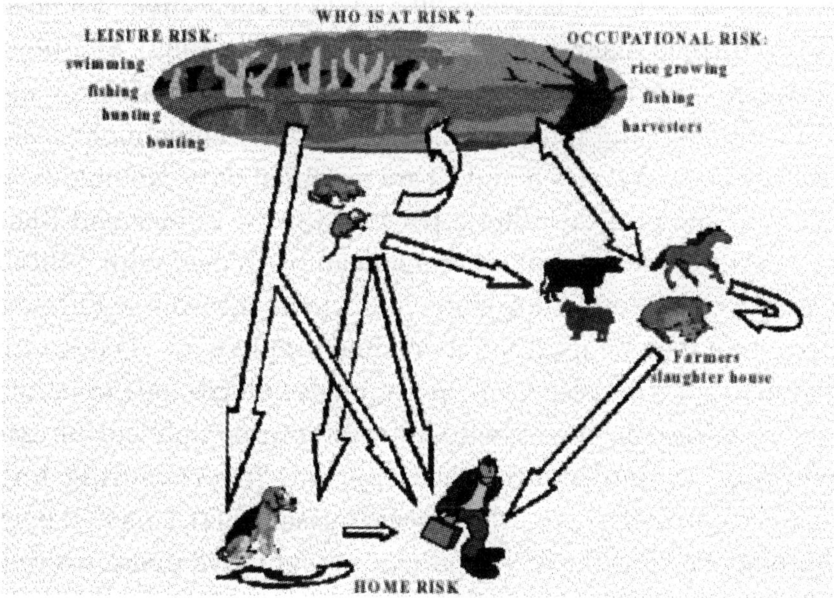

Fig. 27 : Epidemiological cycle of *Leptospira* spp. (http://www.bvs.sld.cu).

Microscopic agglutination test (MAT) is the gold standard test, but it is complicated and less sensitive compared to newer tests like IgM ELISA and SAT. As IgM ELISA and Slide agglutination tests (SAT) are simple, sensitive tests which measure IgM antibodies, they are currently used to diagnose leptospirosis at a very early stage instead of MAT. Single sample is adequate for these two tests. The IgM ELISA test is particularly useful in making an early diagnosis, as it is positive as early as 2 days into illness, a time when the clinical manifestation may be nonspecific. It was found to be 100% sensitive and 93% specific in one study (Kaur *et al.*, 2003). Dot-ELISA and dip-stick methods for detecting IgM antibodies are newer screening methods. Faine has evolved a criteria for diagnosis of leptospirosis on the basis of clinical (A), epidemiological (B) and laboratory data (C) respectively. A presumptive diagnosis of leptospirosis may be made if: (i) Parts A and B score = 26 or more (Part C laboratory report is usually not available before fifth day of illness. Thus, it is mainly a clinical and epidemiologic diagnosis during early part of disease) (ii) Part A+B+C = 25 or more. A score between 20 and 25 is suggestive of a possible but unconfirmed diagnosis of leptospirosis (Faine 1982). Modification on Faine's criteria include local factor like rainfall and newer investigations in the total scoring. As per this, epidemiological and laboratory criteria (Parts B and C) are modified only. No modification is made in the clinical criteria (Part A) (Shiva Kumar and Shareek 2004). Severe leptospirosis in human can be treated with antibiotics like doxycycline. ampicillin, amoxicillin, penicillin and erythromycin. Doxycycline may be used for short time prophylaxis. The control of infection in goats and especially pet animals reduces the risk of human disease, but the existence of wild life reservoirs complicate the disease prevention. Rodent control is important in preventing human infections, particularly in urban areas (Russel 1994). Personal hygiene and protective clothing are important preventative measures in high risk occupations. Gloves and face shields can help in preventing infections while working with infected animals or tissues. Rubber boots can decrease the risk of infection in sewer workers and agricultural workers who come in contact with urine-contaminated water.

7.7. Listeriosis

Listeriosis, caused by *Listeria monocytogenes* (Lm) is transmitted from cattle to human either directly through contact with infected animals or indirectly via milk, cheese or meat (Washington state department of health 2002). Listeriosis in humans is seen primarily in pregnant women, newborns, elderly, and immunosuppressed (*e.g.* transplant recipients or AIDS patients). A small population (5-10 %) may act as asymptomatic carriers harboring the organism in their feces or vagina. Disease in adult humans is commonly of the encephalitic or septicemic/visceral form (Working group on zoonoses 2002). The most common treatment is administration of antibiotics like oxytetracycline or penicillin G. Good hygiene and sanitation on the farm is of utmost importance to prevent the spread of the disease to human population. Whenever possible, people at risk for listeriosis should avoid the consumption of foods associated with listeriosis as mentioned earlier. The risk group also need to adhere strictly to the food label directions for storage and "use by" information. It is virtually impossible to provide Listeria-free food products because *L. monocytogenes* infects many animal species with many infections being inapparent, and most importantly the bacterium can survive and grow at refrigeration temperature levels. Other means of prevention include thoroughly cooking raw meats, proper hygiene during food preparation and consuming only pasteurized dairy products. Humans at risk should also avoid contact with animals that have aborted as well as with aborted materials like placenta and fetuses on the farm. Moreover, livestock and crop producers can also help to control the spread of *L. monocytogenes* by avoiding the use of untreated manure on vegetable crops.

7.8. Ringworm

Ringworm is a skin infection in human that can be transmitted from cattle and the species of importance is *T. verrucosum*. People are infected with ringworm through direct contact with infected animals. In humans, ringworm forms itchy areas on the skin that are round and irritated.

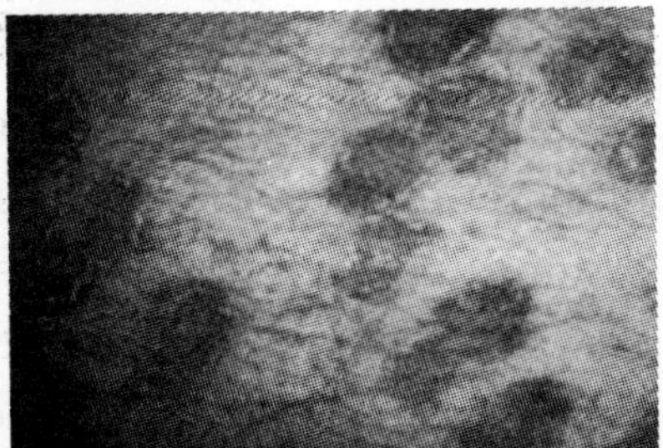

Fig. 28 : Typical ringworm lesion in human patient (http://www.dpi.vic.gov.au)

Treatment helps to limit the spread of the disease to other susceptible person. Topical iodine compounds (5%), chlorhexidine (2%), lime sulphur (2%-5%), and topical antifungal medications are useful for local treatment of lesions. Some severe cases require administration of medications. People treating animals should always wear gloves and protective clothing to prevent from getting this disease (www.ext.vt.edu). Proper cleaning and disinfection of clippers, blankets and other equipment with antiseptic solutions along with good sanitation practices of animal handlers help control the spread of this disease.

7.9. Rabies

People contract rabies through exposure to infected saliva in open wounds or mucous membranes of eyes, nose and mouth. This can occur during examination or treatment of infected cattle. However, other contacts such as petting a rabid animal or contact with the blood, urine or faeces of a rabid animal do not constitute an exposure and is not an indication for prophylaxis (Afshar 1979). After the first exposure, there is acute incubation phase of the disease during which itching and discomfort occur at the site of bite wound. It has a sensation of needle pricking the skin. In addition, the person may develop fever and a headache. These symptoms may last from 2 days to weeks. This is followed by another incubation period. The National Institute of Health (NIH) suggests that the average latent incubation phase may vary from 3 to 7 weeks although a period extending to about 10 years is also reported. Thereafter, there is development of symptoms like anxiety, delirium, drooling of saliva, convulsion, hallucination, loss of sensation in an area of the body, insomnia and swallowing difficulty. When these symptoms develop, the person is likely to die. When people develop clinical rabies, the best treatment is supportive care. Healthcare providers do not generally recommend routine pre-exposure prophylaxis with the rabies vaccine in other situations. Healthcare providers administer pre-exposure prophylaxis with the rabies vaccine for several reasons. First, it simplifies therapy by eliminating the need for human rabies immune globulin (HRIG), and decreases the number of rabies vaccine doses needed. Second, it may enhance immunity in people whose post-exposure rabies treatment might be delayed. Finally, it may provide protection to people with inapparent exposures to rabies. Pre-exposure treatment with the rabies vaccine consists of three doses of rabies vaccine given on days 0, 7, and 21 or 28. Doctors use post-exposure prophylaxis (rabies treatment) with the rabies vaccine for people possibly exposed to a rabid animal. Post-exposure treatment for rabies should begin as soon as possible after an exposure. Physicians should evaluate each possible exposure to rabies and, as necessary, consult with local or state public health officials regarding the need for rabies prophylaxis. Post-exposure rabies treatment consists of a regimen of one dose of rabies immune globulin and five doses of rabies vaccine given over a 28-day period. Rabies immune globulin and the first dose of rabies vaccine should be given as soon as possible after exposure. Additional doses of rabies vaccine should be given on days 3, 7, 14, and 28 after the first vaccination. The rabies vaccine works by stimulating a person's immune system to produce antibodies that neutralize the virus. The person develops a protective immune response before the virus reaches the brain and begins to actively replicate. Older rabies vaccines required painful, daily injections in the abdomen, for up to three weeks, and they could produce severe side effects. Current rabies vaccines are relatively painless and are given in arm. Newer rabies vaccines in use today also cause fewer adverse reactions. Possible side effects of the rabies vaccine can include low-grade fever, pain, redness, swelling or itching at the injection site, headache, nausea, abdominal pain, muscle aches and dizziness (US Department of Health and Human Services 2009). Transmission of the virus in unpasteurised cow's milk is theoretically possible. The risk can be defined better if samples of milk and mammary tissues are collected from rabid animal and assayed for the presence, infectivity and viability of the rabies virus. Regardless of the amount of viavle rabies virus that may be shed in cow's milk, the theoretical risk of transmission of rabies via this route can be eliminated if all dairy products are pasteurized before consumption (National Association of State Public Health Veterinarians 1999).

Rabies can also spread to the existing cattle population from wild life reservoirs. In a cooperative program involving the USDA and the CDC, animals such as raccoons, coyotes, foxes, and skunks are vaccinated orally in certain areas of USA where rabid wildlife are frequently found. The oral rabies vaccine is hidden in a bait of fishmeal or other food. The baits are dropped by airplanes into rural areas and spread by hand in urban and suburban areas. But this approach is not feasible in developing countries like India and further studies are required in this aspect.

7.10. Fascioliasis

Studies carried out in recent years have shown human fascioliasis to be an important public health problem (Chen and Mott 1990). Fascioliasis in human have been reported particularly from the north-eastern part of the country (Narain *et al.*, 1997). Human *F. hepatica* infection is determined by the presence of the intermediate snail hosts, domestic herbivorous animals, climatic conditions and the dietary habits of man. Cattle are considered as the predominant animal reservoir. The mode of transmission is the faecal–oral route. Parasite eggs are passed in the faeces of infected animals or humans, thereby contaminating water where they develop within snails. The snails release mature larvae that attach to vegetation and encyst as metacercariae. A person typically becomes infected by ingesting encysted metacercariae attached to aquatic or semi-aquatic plants. Evidence also indicates that infection may occur by drinking water contaminated with floating metacercariae and by ingesting metacercariae attached to the surface of food or kitchen utensils washed with water contaminated with floated metacercariae. Fascioliasis is a serious medical condition due to the size of the parasite. After an incubation phase lasting days to a couple of months, human fascioliasis can be distinguished by an acute and a chronic phase. The acute phase is characterized by the migration of immature worms through the liver and the symptoms are related to haemorrhage and inflammation and are usually severe, including fever, abdominal pain, respiratory disturbances and skin rashes. The chronic phase starts when the worms reach the bile ducts but in such cases, the symptoms are nonspecific and usually mild. However, progressive inflammation leads to fibrosis and thickening of the walls of the ducts and gallbladder that eventually may result in progressive blockage due to parasites, parasite fragments or debris. In this case, biliary colic pain is a characteristic symptom. Chronic infections may result in biliary cirrhosis with scarring and fibrosis of the liver and growth deficiencies. Ultrasonography in addition to ELISA and Western Blot analysis of the parasitic antigen aid to diagnosis of human fascioliasis. False fasciolosis (pseudofasciolosis) refers to the presence of eggs in the stool not because of an actual infection but due to recent ingestion of infected livers containing eggs. This situation with its potential for misdiagnosis can be avoided by having the patient follow a liver-free diet several days before a repeat stool examination (Hillyer 1999). Single dose of triclabendazole (Fasinax@10 mg/kg body weight) is the most common drug of choice against human fascioliasis. The drug is active against both immature and adult parasites with high cure rates (O'Brien 1998).

References

1. Schrag, S. J. and Wiener, P. (1995). Emerging infectious disease: what are the relative roles of ecology and evolution. *Trends Ecol. Evol.*, 10(8): 319-324.
2. Daszak, P., Cunningham, A. A. and Hyatt, A. D. (2001). Anthropogenic environmental change and the emergence of infectious disease in wildlife. *Acta trop.*, 78(2): 103-116.
3. Dobson, A. and Foufopoulos J. (2001). Emerging infectious pathogens of wildlife. *Philos. Trans. roy. Soc. Lond., B, biol. Sci.*, 356(1411): 1001-1012.
4. United Nations Convention on Biological Diversity (CBD) (2003). Pilot Assessments: the ecological and socioeconomic impact of invasive alien species on island ecosystems. CBD, Montreal, pp. 38. Website: http://www.biodiv.org/doc/ref/alien/ias-inland-en.pdf.

5. Friedlander, A. M. (1999). Clinical aspects, diagnosis and treatment of anthrax. *J. Appl. Microbiol.*, 87: 303.

6. Friedlander, A. M., Welkos, S. L., Pitt, M. L. M., Ezzell, J. W., Worsham, P. L. and Rose, K. J. (1993). Postexposure prophylaxis against experimental inhalation anthrax. *J. Infect. Dis.*, 167: 1239-42.

7. Flores-Castro, R. and Baer, G. M. (1980). Brucellosis (*Brucella melitensis*), Zoonotic implications. *In*: *CRC Handbook series in Zoonoses, Section A: Bacterial, Rickettsial and Mycotic diseases*, CRC Press Inc., Boca Raton, F. L. 195.

8. Bielaszewska, M., Janda, J., Blahova, K., Minarikova, H., Jikova, E., Karmali, M. A., Laubova, J., Sikulova, J., Preston, M. A, Khakhria, R., Karch, H., Klazarova, H. and Nyc, O. (1997). Human *Escherichia coli* O157: H7 infection associated with the consumption of unpasteurized goat's milk. *Am. Pub. Health. Assoc.*, 119: 299-305.

9. Kudva, I. T., Jelacic, S., Tarr, P. I., Youderian, P. and Hovde, C. J. (1999). Biocontrol of *Escerichiacoli* O157 with O157 specific bacteriophages. *Appl. Environ. Microbiol.*, 65(9): 3767-3773.

10. Robinson, D. A. and Jones, D. M. (1981). Milk-borne campylobacter infection. *BMJ.*, 282:1374-1376.

11. Grange, J.M. and Zumla, A. (2002). The global emergency of tuberculosis: what is the cause? *J. Royal Soc. Promot. Health.*, 122(2): 78–81.

12. OIE. (2005). The centre for food security and public health. Leptospirosis. pp 1-9.

13. http://www.bvs.sld.cu.

14. Kaur, I. R., Sachdeva, R., Arora, V. and Talwar, V. (2003). Preliminary survey of leptospirosis among febrile patients from urban slums of East Delhi. *J. Assoc. Physic. Ind.*, 51: 249-51.

15. Faine, S. (1982). Guidelines for the control of leptospirosis. WHO Offset Publication No. 67, Geneva.

16. Shiva Kumar, S. and Shareek, P. S. (2004). Diagnosis of leptospirosis utilizing modified Faine's criteria. *J. Assoc. Physic. Ind.*, 52: 678-679.

17. Russell, L. (1994). Leptospirosis. Scientific meeting for leptospirosis. pp. 5-7.

18. Washington State Department of Health. (2002). Listeriosis. pp. 1-5.

19. Working Group on Zoonoses. (2002). Zoonotic Pathogens: Health Risks from *Listeria*. Federal Veterinary Office Magazine. pp. 14-15.

20. http://www.dpi.vic.gov.au.

21. www.ext.vt.edu.

22. Afshar, A. A. (1979). A review of non-bite transmission of rabies virus infection. *British Vet J.*, 135: 142-148.

23. US Department of Health and Human Services. (2009). Vaccine information statement. Centres for Disease Control and Prevention.

24. National Association of State Public Health Veteriarians, Inc. (1999). Compendium of animal rabies control. *J. Am. Vet. Med. Assoc.*, 214: 198-202.

25. Chen, M.G. and Mott, K.E. (1990). Progress in assessment of morbidity due to *Fasciola hepatica* infection: a review of recent literature. *Trop. Dis. Bull.*, 87: R1–R38.

26. Narain, K., Biswas, D., Rajguru, S. K. and Mahanta, J. (1997). Human distomatosis due to Ffasciola hepatica infection in Assam, India. *J. Commun. Dis.*, 29(2): 161-165.

27. Hillyer, G. V. (1999). Immunodiagnosis of human and animal fascilosis. *In*: Dalton, J. P. *Fasciolosis*. Wallingford, Oxon, U. K. CABI Pub. pp. 435-447.

28. O'Brien, D. J. (1998). Fasciolosis: a threat to livestock. *Irish Vet. J.*, 51: 539–541.

□□□